1006648982

The Top 100 Drug Interactions

A Guide to Patient Management

2010 Edition

Philip D. Hansten, PharmD
Professor Emeritus of Pharmacy
University of Washington
Seattle, Washington

John R. Horn, PharmD
Professor of Pharmacy
University of Washington
Seattle, Washington

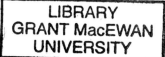

The Top 100 Drug Interactions

A Guide to Patient Management

Published by

H&H Publications, LLP
Box 1418
Freeland, WA 98249-1418
USA

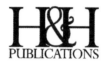

Visit H&H Publications:
www.hanstenandhorn.com

Printed in the United States of America

Publisher's Note

This guide to drug interactions was prepared solely by the authors. It is not intended to replace more complete sources of drug interaction information.

The authors and publisher of this book have made every effort to ensure the accuracy of the information presented. Nevertheless, it is the responsibility of the reader to assess the appropriateness of the recommendations presented after consideration of patient specific factors and after consideration of any new developments in the field. The authors and publisher disclaim all responsibility for any errors or damage incurred as a consequence of the use of the information contained in this book.

Comments or suggestions? Visit our website at www.hanstenandhorn.com.

ISBN: 978-0-9819440-1-2

Table of Contents

Introduction

It is often difficult to distinguish clinically important from unimportant drug interactions. Given the lack of definitive epidemiological studies of drug interactions in patients, it is seldom possible to determine with certainty which interactions actually represent the most danger to public health. This book represents an attempt to identify drug interactions that should not be ignored in clinical practice. The original edition of this book contained about 100 interaction monographs. It has grown substantially and now contains about 5000 individual drug-drug interactions. The interactions are arranged according to *object drug* (the drug affected by the interaction) and *precipitant drug* (the drug causing the interaction). The precipitant drugs are grouped by mechanism (e.g., enzyme inhibitors or enzyme inducers) to show the types of interactions in which each object drug participates. Use the index to find drugs listed by their generic name. This book is intended to be a guide to drug interactions and the reader is reminded to check the cytochrome P450 table (see page 8) for additional drug combinations that may interact.

Information about the use of this book:
- This book employs an operational classification for drug interactions (see description of ORCA system on page 7).
- Note that the magnitude of drug interactions tends to vary widely (usually 6-8-fold or more) between patients and is usually difficult to predict. For that reason, we do not generally provide specific values defining the magnitude of an interaction. Even modest changes in the plasma concentration of drugs with narrow therapeutic ranges, or in patients with certain predisposing factors, can produce severe adverse effects.
- Some interactions, not yet reported in the literature, are included based on the known properties of the two drugs.
- Although it is often desirable to avoid adverse drug interactions by using non-interacting alternatives, few of the interactions in this book represent absolute contraindications. The prescriber is urged to carefully consider the risk-benefit ratio associated with the coadministration of interacting drugs.
- We have attempted to provide non-interacting alternatives for the object and/or precipitant drugs under the Comments or Management Class monograph headings. The prescriber should consider all patient variables before selecting an alternative agent. Drug product labeling should be consulted for full prescribing information.
- For the most part, this book does not include drug interactions with food, smoking, or drugs used primarily during surgery. Neither does it include predictable pharmacologic interactions such as additive CNS or bone marrow depression, renal toxins, or desirable drug-drug interactions.

- Users of this book would benefit from access to a more detailed, referenced drug interaction source such as *Hansten and Horn's Drug Interactions Analysis and Management*. To order *Hansten and Horn's Drug Interactions Analysis and Management* or to obtain information on the mechanisms of drug interactions and access over 75 concise reviews of specific interactions and related topics, visit our website at **www.hanstenandhorn.com**.

New for the 2010 Edition

New monographs for the 2010 Edition involve drugs such as antiarrhythmics, antidepressants, antihypertensives, aprepitant, aripiprazole, eplerenone, linezolid, quetiapine, ranolazine, tyrosine kinase inhibitors, and valproic acid; most existing monographs have been revised. We have retained the book's size that was instituted last year. The CYP450 table has been updated with a number of new entries. Additions and revisions have been made to all of the other tables as well, such as the QT Prolongation table and the Herbal Drug Interaction section.

We are gratified by the response to The Top 100 Drug Interactions since the first edition was published in 2000. More than 300,000 copies of the various editions are in print, and it has been translated into Japanese and Korean. We are pleased that several schools and colleges of pharmacy have adopted the book as a text for drug interaction courses. Substantial student discounts are available. Suggestions and corrections are welcome at www.hanstenandhorn.com.

About the Authors:

Drs. Philip Hansten and John Horn are recognized as international authorities in the field of drug-drug interactions. Their combined experience exceeds 60 years in the field. Most of their scholarship has focused on translational research designed to bring the basic principles of drug interactions into clinical focus. Their drug interaction books have been translated into 6 languages and have sold more than one million copies worldwide since 1971. Hansten and Horn have lectured extensively in North America and in over two-dozen other countries worldwide.

Operational Classification of Drug Interactions

The OpeRational ClassificAtion (ORCA) system for drug interactions used by Hansten and Horn in this book was developed by the Drug Interaction Foundation in an effort to improve the clinical utility of classification systems for drug interactions. (See reference below for more detailed description of ORCA.) As such, the classification system differs from all others in its fundamental approach to evaluation of potential interactions. The system assigns drug interactions to categories based on the *management* of the interaction (which is generally the primary issue confronting the health professional). The objective is to provide a classification system that practitioners will find both easier to use and of greater benefit as a clinical decision support tool than previous classification systems based on estimated "clinical significance" or levels of documentation. **Note: only drug interactions in Classes 1, 2, and 3 are included in this book.**

Class 1:	Avoid Combination (*Risk of combination outweighs benefit*)
Class 2:	Usually Avoid Combination (*Use only under special circumstances*) • Interactions for which there are clearly preferable alternatives for one or both drugs. • Interactions to avoid by using an alternative drug or other therapy unless the benefit is judged to outweigh the increased risk.
Class 3:	Minimize Risk (*Assess risk and take one or more of the following actions if needed*) • *Consider alternatives:* Alternatives may be available that are less likely to interact • *Circumvent:* Take action to minimize the interaction (without avoiding combination.) • *Monitor:* Early detection can minimize the risk of an adverse outcome.
Class 4:	No Special Precautions (*Risk of adverse outcome appears small*)
Class 5:	Ignore (*Evidence suggests that the drugs do not interact*)

Hansten PD, Horn JR, Hazlet TK. ORCA: OpeRational ClassificAtion of Drug Interactions. *J Am Pharm Assoc* 2001;41:161-5.

Cytochrome P450 Enzymes and Transporters Table

Inhibition or induction of cytochrome P450 (CYP450) drug metabolizing isozymes is a relatively common mechanism by which clinically important drug interactions occur. The recommended nomenclature for these enzymes is "CYP" to designate human cytochrome P450, followed by an Arabic number to designate the P450 family, followed by a capital letter to designate the subfamily; followed by an Arabic number to indicate the individual gene. Thus, examples of individual isozymes would include CYP1A2, CYP2C9, CYP2D6, etc. Some important characteristics of CYP450 isozymes include the following:

- Inhibition is substrate independent (e.g., a potent inhibitor of CYP3A4 is very likely to inhibit the metabolism of any drug metabolized by CYP3A4).
- Some (but **not** all) substrates are also inhibitors for the same enzyme, probably due to competitive inhibition of the enzyme (e.g., tacrine and CYP1A2 or verapamil and CYP3A4).
- Some inhibitors affect more than one enzyme or transporter (e.g., amiodarone inhibits CYP2C9, CYP2D6, CYP3A4 and P-glycoprotein.
- The magnitude of inhibition of CYP450 enzymes tends to be dose related over the dosage range of the inhibitor (e.g., cimetidine 1200 mg/day is a more potent inhibitor than 400 mg/day).
- An inhibitor may produce inhibition of one isozyme at one dose, but require a larger dose of the inhibitor to inhibit another CYP isozyme (e.g., fluconazole inhibits CYP2C9 at low doses such as 100 mg/day, but significant inhibition of CYP3A4 requires larger doses such as 200-400 mg/day).
- Some substrates are metabolized by more than one isozyme (e.g., diazepam is metabolized by both CYP2C19 and CYP3A4, and tricyclic antidepressants are metabolized by many CYP450 isozymes).
- Most CYP450 isozyme inhibitors are themselves metabolized by the liver, but some are drugs with primarily renal elimination (e.g., cimetidine, fluconazole).
- Enantiomers may be metabolized by different isozymes. For example, the relatively weak anticoagulant R-warfarin is metabolized primarily by CYP1A2, while the more potent S-warfarin is metabolized primarily by CYP2C9. Thus, inhibitors of CYP1A2 tend to produce only small increases in the hypoprothrombinemic response to warfarin, while CYP2C9 inhibitors can produce large increases in warfarin effect.

Drug transporters are also involved in many drug interactions. These transporters (also called ABC transporters) are found in many tissues, and they actively pump drug molecules either out of cells (efflux) or into cells (uptake). Many of the characteristics of CYP450 isozymes (above) apply to transporters as well. We have included P-glycoprotein (PGP), one of the most important transporters for drug interactions, as a column in the following table—two other transporters (OCT and OAT) are included in the "Misc" column on the table.

Legend:

⊙ = Substrate for isozyme ↓ = Inhibitor (weak inhibitors = ↓) ↑ = Inducer (weak inducer = ↑) * = Primary metabolic path for drugs with multiple pathways	<u>Miscellaneous Column</u>: 1 = CYP2B6 substrate 2 = CYP2B6 inhibitor 3 = CYP2C8 substrate 4 = CYP2C8 inhibitor 5 = OCT substrate 6 = OCT inhibitor 7 = OAT/OATP substrate 8 = OAT/OATP inhibitor

Drug	1A2	2C9	2C19	2D6	3A4	PGP	Misc
Alcohol (intoxicating dose)[1]		↓					
Alfentanil (Alfenta)					⊙	⊙↓	
Alfuzosin (Uroxatral)					⊙		
Aliskiren (Tekturna)					⊙		
Almotriptan (Axert)				⊙	⊙		
Alosetron (Lotronex)	⊙	⊙			⊙		
Alprazolam (Xanax)					⊙		
Alprenolol				⊙			
Ambrisentan (Letairis)			⊙		⊙	⊙	
Amiodarone (Cordarone)		↓		↓	⊙↓	↓	3,5
Amitriptyline (Elavil)	⊙		⊙	⊙*	⊙	⊙	
Aminoglutethimide		↑			↑		
Amlodipine (Norvasc)					⊙		
Amprenavir (Agenerase)		⊙		⊙	⊙*↓	⊙	
Anagrelide (Agrylin)	⊙						
Aprepitant (Emend)	⊙	↑	⊙		⊙*↓		
Aripiprazole (Abilify)[2]				⊙	⊙		
Artemisinin	↓		↑				
Astemizole					⊙		
Atazanavir (Reyataz)	↓				⊙↓		
Atomoxetine (Strattera)				⊙			
Atorvastatin (Lipitor)					⊙	⊙	7,8
Azapropazone		⊙					
Azithromycin (Zithromax)						⊙↓	
Barbiturates	↑	↑	↑		↑	↑	

Drug	1A2	2C9	2C19	2D6	3A4	PGP	Misc
Basiliximab					↓		
Bendamustine (Treanda)	⊙						
Bepridil (Vascor)					⊙	↓	
Bexarotene (Targretin)					⊙↑		
Bortezomib (Velcade)	⊙		⊙		⊙*		
Bosentan (Tracleer)		⊙↑			⊙↑		7
Bromocriptine (Parlodel)					⊙		
Budesonide (Entocort)					⊙	⊙	
Bupivacaine (Sensorcaine)					⊙		
Buprenophine (Subutex)					⊙		
Bupropion (Wellbutrin)				↓			1
Buspirone (Buspar)					⊙		
Caffeine	⊙						
Candesartan (Atacand)		⊙					
Capecitabine (Xeloda)		↓					
Carbamazepine (Tegretol)	↑	↑			⊙↑	↑	3
Carisoprodol (Soma)			⊙				
Carvedilol (Coreg)				⊙		⊙	
Celecoxib (Celebrex)		⊙		↓			
Cetirizine (Zyrtec)						⊙	
Cevimeline (Evoxac)				⊙	⊙		
Chloramphenicol			↓		↓		
Chloroquine (Aralen)				↓			3
Chlorpheniramine				⊙↓	⊙		
Chlorpromazine (Thorazine)				⊙↓			
Chlorpropamide (Diabinese)		⊙					
Cilostazol (Pletal)			⊙		⊙		
Cimetidine (Tagamet)	↓		↓	↓			5,6,8
Cinacalcet (Sensipar)	⊙			⊙↓	⊙		
Ciprofloxacin (Cipro)	↓						
Cisapride (Propulsid)					⊙		
Citalopram (Celexa)			⊙*	⊙↓	⊙	⊙	
Clarithromycin (Biaxin)					⊙↓	↓	
Clomipramine (Anafranil)	⊙		⊙	⊙*	⊙		
Clonazepam (Klonopin)					⊙		3

Drug	1A2	2C9	2C19	2D6	3A4	PGP	Misc
Clopidogrel (Plavix)		↓	↓⊙*		⊙		2
Clozapine (Clozaril)[3]	⊙*		⊙	⊙	⊙		
Codeine				⊙			
Colchicine					⊙	⊙	
Conivaptan (Vaprisol)					⊙↓	↓	
Co-trimoxazole (Septra)		⊙↓			⊙		4
Cyclobenzaprine (Flexeril)	⊙				⊙		
Cyclophosphamide (Cytoxan)					⊙		2
Cyclosporine (Neoral)					⊙↓	⊙↓	8
Danazol (Danocrine)					↓		
Dapsone (Avlosulfon)					⊙		
Darifenacin (Enablex)				⊙	⊙		
Darunavir (Prezista)					⊙↓		
Dasatinib (Sprycel)					⊙↓		
Daunorubicin (Cerubidine)						⊙	
Debrisoquin				⊙			
Delavirdine (Rescriptor)		↓	↓		⊙↓		
Desipramine (Norpramin)			⊙	⊙*			
Deslansoprazole (Kapidex)			⊙		⊙		
Desloratadine (Clarinex)					⊙		
Desvenlafaxine (Pristiq)				↓	⊙		
Dexamethasone (Decadron)					⊙↑	⊙	
Dextromethorphan				⊙*	⊙		
Diazepam (Valium)			⊙*		⊙		
Diclofenac (Voltaren)		⊙			⊙		
Digoxin (Lanoxin)						⊙	
Dihydrocodeine				⊙			
Dihydroergotamine					⊙		
Diltiazem (Cardizem)					⊙↓	⊙↓	
Diphenhydramine (Benadryl)	⊙		⊙	⊙*↓			
Disopyramide (Norpace)					⊙		6
Disulfiram (Antabuse)		↓					
Docetaxel (Taxotere)					⊙	⊙	
Dofetilide (Tikosyn)					⊙		5
Dolasetron (Anzemet)				⊙*	⊙		

Drug	1A2	2C9	2C19	2D6	3A4	PGP	Misc
Donepezil (Aricept)				⊙	⊙*		
Doxepin (Sinequan)		⊙	⊙	⊙*			
Doxorubicin (Adriamycin)					⊙	⊙	
Doxifluridine		↓					
Dronabinol (Marinol)		⊙					
Dronedarone (Multaq)				↓	⊙↓	↓	
Droperidol (Inapsine)					⊙	⊙	
Duloxetine (Cymbalta)	⊙			⊙↓			
Dutasteride (Avodart)					⊙		
Ebastine (Kestine)					⊙		
Efavirenz (Sustiva)		↓	↓		⊙↑		1
Eletriptan (Relpax)					⊙	⊙	
Encainide				⊙			
Enoxacin (Penetrex)	↓						
Eplerenone (Inspra)					⊙		
Ergotamine (Ergomar)					⊙		
Erlotinib (Tarceva)	⊙				⊙*		
Erythromycin (E-Mycin)					⊙↓	⊙↓	
Escitalopram (Lexapro)			⊙*	⊙↓	⊙		
Esomeprazole (Nexium)			⊙*↓		⊙		
Estazolam (Prosom)					⊙		
Eszopiclone (Lunesta)					⊙		
Ethinyl Estradiol	↓				⊙↓	⊙	
Ethosuximide (Zarontin)					⊙		
Etoposide (Vepesid)					⊙	⊙	
Etravirine (Intelence)		⊙↓	⊙↓		⊙↑		
Everolimus (Afinitor)					⊙	⊙	
Exemestane (Aromasin)					⊙		
Felbamate (Felbatol)			↓				
Felodipine (Plendil)					⊙		
Fenofibrate (Tricor)						↓	
Fentanyl (Sublimaze)					⊙	⊙	
Fesoterodine (Toviaz)				⊙	⊙*		
Fexofenadine (Allegra)						⊙	7
Finasteride (Proscar)					⊙		

Drug	1A2	2C9	2C19	2D6	3A4	PGP	Misc
Flecainide (Tambocor)				⊙↓			
Fluconazole (Diflucan)[4]		↓	↓		↓		
Fluorouracil (5-FU)		↓					
Fluoxetine (Prozac)[5]		⊙↓	⊙↓	⊙*↓	↓		
Flurazepam (Dalmane)					⊙		
Flurbiprofen (Ansaid)		⊙					
Flutamide (Eulexin)	⊙						
Fluvastatin (Lescol)		⊙↓					
Fluvoxamine	⊙↓	↓	↓	⊙*↓	↓		
Fosamprenavir (Lexiva)					⊙↓		
Frovatriptan (Frova)	⊙						
Galantamine (Reminyl)				⊙	⊙*		
Gefitinib (Iressa)				⊙	⊙		
Gemfibrozil (Lopid)		↓					4
Glimepiride (Amaryl)		⊙					
Glipizide (Glucotrol)		⊙					
Glyburide (DiaBeta)		⊙				⊙	
Granisetron (Kytril)					⊙		
Grapefruit[6]					↓	↓	8
Griseofulvin (Grisactin)		↑			↑		
Halofantrine (Halfan)				↓	⊙		
Haloperidol (Haldol)				⊙*↓	⊙		
Hydrocodone (Vicodin)				⊙			
Hydroxychloroquine				↓			
Ibuprofen (Advil, Motrin)		⊙					3
Ifosfamide (Ifex)					⊙		1
Iloperidone (Fanapt)				⊙	⊙		
Imatinib (Gleevec)		↓		↓	⊙↓	⊙	
Imipramine (Tofranil)	⊙		⊙	⊙*	⊙		
Indinavir (Crixivan)					⊙↓	⊙↓	
Indiplon	⊙				⊙		
Indomethacin (Indocin)		⊙					
Interleukin-10					↓		
Irbesartan (Avapro)		⊙					
Irinotecan (Camptosar)					⊙	⊙	

Drug	1A2	2C9	2C19	2D6	3A4	PGP	Misc
Isoniazid (INH, Nydrazid)			↓		↓		
Isradipine (DynaCirc)					⊙		
Itraconazole (Sporanox)					⊙↓	↓	
Ivabradine					⊙		
Ixabepilone (Ixempra)					⊙		
Ketoconazole (Nizoral)					⊙↓	↓	
Lacosamide (Vimpat)			⊙				
Lapatinib (Tykerb)					⊙↓	↓	
Lansoprazole (Prevacid)			⊙		⊙		
Leflunomide (Arava)		↓					
Levofloxacin (Maxaquin)							6
Levomethadyl (Orlaam)					⊙		
Lidocaine	⊙*				⊙		
Loperamide (Imodium)					⊙	⊙	3
Lopinavir (Kaletra)					⊙		
Loratadine (Claritin)				⊙	⊙*	⊙	
Losartan (Cozaar)[7]		⊙*			⊙		
Lovastatin (Mevacor)					⊙*	⊙	
Maprotiline (Ludiomil)				⊙			
Maraviroc (Selzentry)					⊙	⊙	
Mefloquine (Lariam)					⊙	⊙↓	
Melatonin	⊙*	⊙					
Meloxicam (Mobic)		⊙*			⊙		
Mephenytoin (Mesantoin)			⊙				
Meropenem (Merrem)							7
Mesoridazine (Serentil)				⊙			
Metformin (Glucophage)							5
Methadone			⊙	⊙		⊙?	1
Methamphetamine				⊙			
Methotrexate							7
Methylprednisolone					⊙	⊙	
Metoclopramide (Reglan)				⊙			
Metoprolol (Lopressor)				⊙			
Metronidazole (Flagyl)		↓					
Mexiletine (Mexitil)	⊙↓			⊙*			

14

Drug	1A2	2C9	2C19	2D6	3A4	PGP	Misc
Mianserin				⊙			
Miconazole (Monistat)		↓			↓		
Midazolam (Versed)					⊙		
Mifepristone (Mifeprex)					⊙↓	↓	
Mirtazapine (Remeron)	⊙			⊙	⊙		
Mitomycin						⊙	
Moclobemide (Manerix)			⊙↓	↓			
Modafinil (Provigil)[8]		↓	↓		⊙↑		
Montelukast (Singulair)		⊙			⊙		4
Morphine						⊙	
Nafcillin (Unipen)		↑?			↑		
Naproxen (Naprosyn)		⊙					
Nefazodone					⊙↓		
Nateglinide (Starlix)		⊙*			⊙		
Nebivolol (Bystolic)				⊙			
Nelfinavir (Viracept)[9]			⊙		⊙↓	⊙↓	
Nevirapine (Viramune)					⊙↑		1
Nicardipine (Cardene)					⊙↓	↓	
Nifedipine (Adalat)					⊙	↓	
Nilotinib (Tasigna)					⊙↓	⊙	
Nimodipine (Nimotop)					⊙		
Nisoldipine (Sular)					⊙		
Nitrendipine (Baypress)					⊙		
Norfloxacin (Norflox)	↓						
Nortriptyline (Pamelor)				⊙*	⊙	⊙	
Olanzapine (Zyprexa)	⊙*			⊙	⊙	⊙	
Omeprazole (Prilosec)			⊙*↓		⊙		
Ondansetron (Zofran)	⊙*			⊙	⊙	⊙	
Oxcarbazepine (Trileptal)			↓		↑		
Oxybutynin (Ditropan)					⊙		
Oxycodone (Percodan)				⊙	⊙*		
Paclitaxel (Taxol)					⊙	⊙	3
Paliperidone (Invega)				⊙		⊙	
Palonosetron (Aloxi)	⊙			⊙*	⊙		
Pantoprazole (Protonix)			⊙*		⊙		

15

Drug	1A2	2C9	2C19	2D6	3A4	PGP	Misc
Paricalcitol (Zemplar)					⊙		
Paroxetine (Paxil)				⊙↓		⊙	
Parsugrel (Effient)		⊙	⊙		⊙		1
Pazopanib (Votrient)				↓	⊙↓		
Pentamidine (Pentam)			⊙				
Perhexiline (Pexid)				⊙			
Perphenazine (Trilafon)				⊙↓			
Phenobarbital	↑	⊙↑	⊙↑		↑		
Phenytoin (Dilantin)	↑	⊙*↓	⊙↑		↑		
Pimozide (Orap)	⊙				⊙*		
Pioglitazone (Actos)					⊙		3
Piroxicam (Feldene)		⊙					
Plicamycin (Mithracin)						⊙	
Posaconazole (Noxafil)					↓	⊙↓	
Pravastatin (Pravachol)							7
Praziquantel (Biltricide)					⊙		
Prednisolone					⊙		
Prednisone					⊙	⊙	
Primidone (Mysoline)	↑	↑	↑		↑		
Probenecid (Benemid)							7,8
Proguanil (active metabolite)			⊙				
Procainamide (Procan)							5
Promethazine (Phenergan)				⊙↓			
Propafenone (Rythmol)	⊙			⊙*↓	⊙	↓	
Propoxyphene (Darvon)				⊙↓	⊙*↓		
Propranolol (Inderal)			⊙	⊙*			
Protriptyline (Vivactil)				⊙			
Quazepam (Doral)					⊙		
Quetiapine (Seroquel)					⊙		
Quinacrine				↓	⊙		
Quinidine (Quinidex)				↓	⊙	⊙↓	5,6
Quinine				↓	⊙		
Quinupristin (Synercid)					↓		
Rabeprazole (Aciphex)			⊙				
Ramelteon (Rozerem)	⊙*	⊙			⊙		

Drug	1A2	2C9	2C19	2D6	3A4	PGP	Misc
Ranolazine (Ranexa)				⊙↓	⊙*↓	⊙↓	
Rasagiline (Azilect)	⊙						
Repaglinide (Prandin)					⊙		3
Rifabutin (Mycobutin)					⊙↑		
Rifampin (Rimactane)	↑	↑	↑	↑	↑	⊙↑	
Rifapentine (Priftin)		↑			↑		
Risperidone (Risperdal)				⊙*↓	⊙	⊙	
Ritonavir (Norvir)[10]				↓?	⊙↓	⊙↓	
Ropinirole (Requip)	⊙						
Ropivacaine (Naropin)	⊙*				⊙		
Rosiglitazone (Avandia)		⊙					3
Rosuvastatin (Crestor)		⊙					7
Salmeterol (Serevent)					⊙		
Saquinavir (Invirase)					⊙↓	⊙↓	
Saxagliptin (Onglyza)					⊙		
Selegiline (Eldepryl)	⊙				⊙		1
Sertindole (Serlect)				⊙	⊙		
Sertraline (Zoloft)			⊙*	⊙↓	⊙	⊙	
Sibutramine (Meridia)					⊙		
Sildenafil (Viagra)		⊙			⊙*		
Silodosin (Rapaflo)					⊙	⊙	
Simvastatin (Zocor)				⊙	⊙*		
Sirolimus (Rapammune)					⊙	⊙	
Sitaxsentan (Thelin)		⊙↓			⊙		
Smoking	↑						
Solifenacin (Vesicare)					⊙		
Sorafenib (Nexavar)					⊙		
St. John's Wort[11]			↑		↑	↑	
Sufentanil (Sufenta)					⊙		
Sulfamethizole		↓					
Sulfamethoxazole (Bactrim)		⊙*↓			⊙		
Sulfaphenazole		↓					
Sulfinpyrazone (Anturane)		↓					
Sunitinib (Sutent)					⊙		
Tacrine (Cognex)	⊙↓						

Drug	1A2	2C9	2C19	2D6	3A4	PGP	Misc
Tacrolimus (Prograf)					⊙	⊙↓	
Tadalafil (Cialis)					⊙		
Tamoxifen (Nolvadex)[12]		↓		⊙	⊙*↓	↓	
Tamsulosin (Flomax)				⊙	⊙		
Telithromycin (Ketek)					↓	↓?	
Temsirolimus (Torisel)					⊙		
Teniposide (Vumon)					⊙	⊙	
Terbinafine (Lamisil)				↓			
Terfenadine					⊙	⊙	
Testosterone					⊙	↓	
Thalidomide (Thalomid)			⊙				
Theophylline	⊙*				⊙		
Thiabendazole (Mintezol)	⊙↓						
Thioridazine (Mellaril)	⊙			⊙*↓	⊙		
Tiagabine (Gabitril)					⊙		
Ticlopidine (Ticlid)			↓				2
Timolol (Blocadren)				⊙			
Tinidazole (Tindamax)					⊙		
Tipranavir (Aptivus)					⊙	⊙↑	
Tizanidine (Zanaflex)	⊙						
Tolbutamide (Orinase)		⊙					
Tolterodine (Detrol)				⊙*	⊙		
Tolvaptan (Samsca)					⊙	⊙	
Topiramate (Topamax)			↓		⊙↑		
Torsemide (Demadex)		⊙					
Tramadol (Ultram)				⊙*	⊙		
Trazodone (Desyrel)				⊙*	⊙		
Triamterene (Dyrenium)	⊙*				⊙		
Triazolam (Halcion)					⊙		
Trimethoprim (Septra)							4
Troleandomycin (TAO)					↓		
Valdecoxib (Bextra)		⊙			⊙		
Valproic Acid (Depakote)		↓					
Valsartan (Diovan)		⊙					
Vardenafil (Levitra)					⊙		

18

Drug	1A2	2C9	2C19	2D6	3A4	PGP	Misc
Venlafaxine (Effexor)				⊙*	⊙	⊙	
Verapamil (Calan)					⊙↓	⊙↓	5,6
Vesnarinone					⊙		
Vinblastine (Velban)					⊙	⊙	
Vincristine (Oncovin)					⊙	⊙	
Vinorelbine (Navelbine)					⊙	⊙	
Voriconazole (Vfend)		⊙↓	⊙↓		⊙↓		
R-Warfarin (Coumadin)	⊙		⊙		⊙		
S-Warfarin (Coumadin)		⊙					
Yohimbine				⊙	⊙		
Zafirlukast (Accolate)	⊙↓	↓			↓		
Zaleplon (Sonata)					⊙		
Zileuton (Zyflo)	⊙↓						
Ziprasidone (Geodon)[13]					⊙		
Zolmitriptan (Zolmig)	⊙						
Zolpidem (Ambien)		⊙			⊙*		
Zonisamide (Zonegran)					⊙		
Zopiclone (Imovane)					⊙		3

Footnotes for Cytochrome P450 Enzymes & Transporters Table

1. Chronic alcohol abuse can result in increased CYP2C9 activity.
2. Aripiprazole is metabolized to an active metabolite, dehydroaripiprazole.
3. The role of CYP3A4 in clozapine metabolism is controversial. Clozapine does not appear to interact with itraconazole or grapefruit juice.
4. Fluconazole inhibition of CYP3A4 is dose related; 100 mg/day usually has little effect, but CYP3A4 inhibition occurs at 200 to 400 mg/day or more, depending on the substrate.
5. Fluoxetine's major metabolite (norfluoxetine) has a very long half-life and is also a potent inhibitor of CYP2D6; thus, CYP2D6 inhibition may persist for several weeks after stopping fluoxetine.

6. The inhibitory effect of grapefruit juice (GFJ) on CYP3A4 is dose related. A single glass of GFJ produces modest CYP3A4 inhibition while multiple glasses daily for several days can produce marked inhibition of CYP3A4. GFJ appears to affect only gut wall CYP3A4, but some effect on hepatic CYP3A4 has not been ruled out.

7. CYP2C9 converts losartan to an active metabolite.

8. Induction of CYP3A4 by modafinil appears to be more intestinal than hepatic.

9. Nelfinavir has been reported to decrease serum concentrations of methadone and ethinyl estradiol, suggesting that it might act as a CYP3A4 inducer in some situations.

10. Long-term ritonavir can induce CYP3A4 and possibly CYP1A2, CYP2C9, and P-glycoprotein. Ritonavir may induce CYP2B6 more rapidly.

11. St. John's wort may also induce other CYP450 isozymes such as CYP2C9, but more clinical data are needed. Single dose St. John's wort may inhibit P-glycoprotein.

12. Tamoxifen is predominantly metabolized by CYP3A4 to inactive metabolites, but CYP2D6 is responsible for converting tamoxifen to active metabolites.

13. About one-third of ziprasidone is metabolized by CYP3A4 and about two-thirds is metabolized by aldehyde oxidase.

OBJECT DRUGS	PRECIPITANT DRUGS	
Acetaminophen (Tylenol)	**Enzyme Inducers:**	
	Alcohol (Chronic, excessive)	**Phenytoin** (Dilantin)
	Barbiturates	**Primidone** (Mysoline)
	Carbamazepine (Tegretol)	**Rifabutin** (Mycobutin)
	Efavirenz (Sustiva)	**Rifampin** (Rifadin)
	Isoniazid (INH)	**Rifapentine** (Priftin)
	Nevirapine (Viramune)	**St. John's Wort**
	Oxcarbazepine (Trileptal)	

COMMENTS: Enzyme inducers have been reported to increase the formation of a toxic acetaminophen metabolite, thus increasing the risk of hepatotoxicity in patients taking overdoses of acetaminophen (or large and/or prolonged therapeutic doses). The analgesic effect of acetaminophen may also be reduced by enzyme inducers due to enhanced acetaminophen metabolism. There is debate about whether chronic excessive alcohol use increases the risk of acetaminophen toxicity, but caution is advised pending more data. Isoniazid has a biphasic effect, first reducing and then increasing toxic metabolite formation.

MANAGEMENT CLASS 3: ASSESS RISK & TAKE ACTION IF NECESSARY

- *Circumvent/Minimize*: Patients on enzyme inducers (or who regularly have 3 or more daily drinks of alcohol) should avoid prolonged use of large therapeutic doses of acetaminophen. A safe amount of acetaminophen for such patients is not established, but it would be prudent to limit intake of acetaminophen to 2 g/day or less.
- *Consider Alternative*: Since acetaminophen analgesia may be reduced, doses considered safe may be ineffective. Thus, it may be necessary to use alternative analgesics. Note, however, that **salicylates** and **NSAIDs** may produce additive toxicity with excessive alcohol intake.

OBJECT DRUGS	PRECIPITANT DRUGS	
Alfuzosin (Uroxatral)	**Antimicrobials:**	
	Clarithromycin (Biaxin)	**Posaconazole** (Noxafil)
	Erythromycin (E-Mycin)	**Quinupristin** (Synercid)
	Fluconazole (Diflucan)	**Telithromycin** (Ketek)
	Itraconazole (Sporanox)	**Troleandomycin** (TAO)
	Ketoconazole (Nizoral)	**Voriconazole** (Vfend)

COMMENTS: Alfuzosin is primarily metabolized by CYP3A4, and these antimicrobial agents are inhibitors of CYP3A4. Based on a more than 3-fold increase in alfuzosin AUC with ketoconazole, the alfuzosin labeling states that combined use of alfuzosin with potent CYP3A4 inhibitors is contraindicated. Although not all of these antimicrobials have equal potency as CYP3A4 inhibitors, they all would be expected to produce substantial increases in alfuzosin plasma concentrations.

CLASS 2: USE ONLY IF BENEFIT FELT TO OUTWEIGH RISK

- *Use Alternative*:

  Azole Antifungals: Fluconazole appears to be a less potent inhibitor of CYP3A4 than itraconazole or ketoconazole, but in larger doses it also inhibits CYP3A4. **Terbinafine** (Lamisil) does not appear to affect CYP3A4.

- *Monitor*: If alfuzosin is used with a CYP3A4 inhibitor, monitor blood pressure for evidence of hypotension. Placing the patient in the supine position or additional measures (intravenous fluids, vasopressors) may be necessary if hypotension occurs.

OBJECT DRUGS	PRECIPITANT DRUGS	
Alfuzosin (Uroxatral)	**Enzyme Inhibitors:**	
	Amiodarone (Cordarone)	**Diltiazem** (Cardizem)
	Amprenavir (Agenerase)	**Grapefruit**
	Aprepitant (Emend)	**Indinavir** (Crixivan)
	Atazanavir (Reyataz)	**Nelfinavir** (Viracept)
	Conivaptan (Vaprisol)	**Ritonavir** (Norvir)
	Cyclosporine (Neoral)	**Saquinavir** (Invirase)
	Darunavir (Prezista)	**Verapamil** (Isoptin)
	Delavirdine (Rescriptor)	

COMMENTS: Alfuzosin is primarily metabolized by CYP3A4, and these agents are inhibitors of CYP3A4. The alfuzosin labeling states that combined use of alfuzosin with potent CYP3A4 inhibitors is contraindicated. Although not all of these antimicrobials have equal potency as CYP3A4 inhibitors, they all would be expected to produce substantial increases in alfuzosin plasma concentrations.

CLASS 2: USE ONLY IF BENEFIT FELT TO OUTWEIGH RISK

- *Use Alternative*:

  Calcium Channel Blockers: Calcium channel blockers other than diltiazem and verapamil are unlikely to significantly inhibit the metabolism of alfuzosin.
  Grapefruit: Orange juice does not appear to inhibit CYP3A4.

- *Monitor*: If alfuzosin is used with a CYP3A4 inhibitor, monitor blood pressure for evidence of hypotension. Placing the patient in the supine position or additional measures (intravenous fluids, vasopressors) may be necessary if hypotension occurs.

OBJECT DRUGS	PRECIPITANT DRUGS	
Antiarrhythmics	**Antimicrobials:**	
(CYP3A4 Substrates):	**Clarithromycin** (Biaxin)	**Posaconazole** (Noxafil)
Amiodarone (Cordarone)	**Erythromycin** (E-Mycin)	**Quinupristin** (Synercid)
Disopyramide (Norpace)	**Fluconazole** (Diflucan)	**Telithromycin** (Ketek)
Dronedarone (Multaq)	**Itraconazole** (Sporanox)	**Troleandomycin** (TAO)
Quinidine (Quinidex)	**Ketoconazole** (Nizoral)	**Voriconazole** (Vfend)

COMMENTS: Although data are limited, any CYP3A4 inhibitor could increase the plasma concentrations of amiodarone, disopyramide, or quinidine. Toxicity including cardiac arrhythmias could result. Assume that all CYP3A4 inhibitors interact until proven otherwise.

CLASS 3: ASSESS RISK & TAKE ACTION IF NECESSARY

- *Consider Alternative*:
  Azole Antifungals: Fluconazole appears to be a less potent inhibitor of CYP3A4 than itraconazole or ketoconazole, but in larger doses it also inhibits CYP3A4. **Terbinafine** (Lamisil) does not appear to affect CYP3A4.
  Macrolide Antibiotics: Unlike erythromycin, clarithromycin and troleandomycin, other macrolides such as **azithromycin** (Zithromax) and **dirithromycin*** do not appear to inhibit CYP3A4. (*not available in US)
- *Monitor*: Monitor for altered antiarrhythmic response if the CYP3A4 inhibitor is initiated, discontinued, or changed in dosage. Monitor for ECG changes indicating antiarrhythmic toxicity, and measure antiarrhythmic plasma concentrations as needed.

OBJECT DRUGS	PRECIPITANT DRUGS
Antiarrhythmics	**Antidepressants:**
(CYP3A4 Substrates):	**Fluvoxamine** (Luvox)
Amiodarone (Cordarone)	**Nefazodone**
Disopyramide (Norpace)	
Dronedarone (Multaq)	
Quinidine (Quinidex)	

COMMENTS: Although data are limited, antidepressants that inhibit CYP3A4 could increase the plasma concentrations of amiodarone, disopyramide, or quinidine. Toxicity including cardiac arrhythmias could result. Assume that all CYP3A4 inhibitors interact until proven otherwise.

CLASS 3: ASSESS RISK & TAKE ACTION IF NECESSARY

- *Consider Alternative*:
  Antidepressants: **Citalopram** (Celexa), **desvenlafaxine** (Pristiq), **paroxetine** (Paxil), **sertraline** (Zoloft), and **venlafaxine** (Effexor) appear to have minimal effects on CYP3A4. **Fluoxetine** (Prozac) appears to be a weak inhibitor of CYP3A4.
- *Monitor*: Monitor for altered antiarrhythmic response if the CYP3A4 inhibitor is initiated, discontinued, or changed in dosage. Monitor for ECG changes indicating antiarrhythmic toxicity, and measure antiarrhythmic plasma concentrations as needed.

OBJECT DRUGS	PRECIPITANT DRUGS
Antiarrhythmics (CYP3A4 Substrates):	**Calcium Channel Blockers:**
Amiodarone (Cordarone)	**Diltiazem** (Cardizem)
Disopyramide (Norpace)	**Verapamil** (Isoptin)
Dronedarone (Multaq)	
Quinidine (Quinidex)	

COMMENTS: Although data are limited, any calcium channel blocker that inhibits CYP3A4 could increase the plasma concentrations of amiodarone, disopyramide, dronedarone, or quinidine. Toxicity including cardiac arrhythmias could result. Assume that all CYP3A4 inhibitors interact until proven otherwise.

CLASS 3: ASSESS RISK & TAKE ACTION IF NECESSARY
- ***Consider Alternative*:**
  Calcium Channel Blockers: Calcium channel blockers other than diltiazem and verapamil are unlikely to inhibit the metabolism of these antiarrhythmics.
- ***Monitor*:** Monitor for altered antiarrhythmic response if the CYP3A4 inhibitor is initiated, discontinued, or changed in dosage. Monitor for ECG changes indicating antiarrhythmic toxicity, and measure antiarrhythmic plasma concentrations as needed.

OBJECT DRUGS	PRECIPITANT DRUGS	
Antiarrhythmics	**Enzyme Inhibitors**	
(CYP3A4 Substrates):	**Amiodarone** (Cordarone)	**Delavirdine** (Rescriptor)
Amiodarone (Cordarone)	**Amprenavir** (Agenerase)	**Grapefruit**
Disopyramide (Norpace)	**Aprepitant** (Emend)	**Indinavir** (Crixivan)
Dronedarone (Multaq)	**Atazanavir** (Reyataz)	**Nelfinavir** (Viracept)
Quinidine (Quinidex)	**Conivaptan** (Vaprisol)	**Ritonavir** (Norvir)
	Cyclosporine (Neoral)	**Saquinavir** (Invirase)
	Darunavir (Prezista)	

COMMENTS: Although data are limited, any CYP3A4 inhibitor could increase the plasma concentrations of amiodarone, disopyramide, dronedarone, or quinidine. Toxicity including cardiac arrhythmias could result. Assume that all CYP3A4 inhibitors interact until proven otherwise.

CLASS 3: ASSESS RISK & TAKE ACTION IF NECESSARY
- ***Consider Alternative*:**
  Grapefruit: Orange juice does not appear to inhibit CYP3A4.
- ***Monitor*:** Monitor for altered antiarrhythmic response if the CYP3A4 inhibitor is initiated, discontinued, or changed in dosage. Monitor for ECG changes indicating antiarrhythmic toxicity, and measure antiarrhythmic plasma concentrations as needed.

OBJECT DRUGS	PRECIPITANT DRUGS	
Antiarrhythmics	**Enzyme Inducers:**	
(CYP3A4 Substrates):	**Barbiturates**	**Primidone** (Mysoline)
Amiodarone (Cordarone)	**Carbamazepine** (Tegretol)	**Rifabutin** (Mycobutin)
Disopyramide (Norpace)	**Efavirenz** (Sustiva)	**Rifampin** (Rifadin)
Dronedarone (Multaq)	**Nevirapine** (Viramune)	**Rifapentine** (Priftin)
Quinidine (Quinidex)	**Oxcarbazepine** (Trileptal)	**St. John's Wort**
	Phenytoin (Dilantin)	

COMMENTS: CYP3A4 is quite sensitive to enzyme induction, and enzyme inducers have been shown to reduce plasma concentrations of amiodarone, disopyramide, dronedarone, and quinidine. Depending on the potency of the enzyme inducer, the reductions in antiarrhythmic plasma concentrations may result in substantial reductions in antiarrhythmic effects.

CLASS 3: ASSESS RISK & TAKE ACTION IF NECESSARY

- *Consider Alternative*:

  St. John's Wort: Given the limited evidence of efficacy, St. John's Wort should generally be avoided in patients taking one of these antiarrhythmic agents.

- *Monitor*: Monitor for altered antiarrhythmic response if the CYP3A4 inducer is initiated, discontinued, or changed in dosage. Monitor for ECG changes indicating antiarrhythmic toxicity, and measure antiarrhythmic plasma concentrations as needed. Note that the effect of enzyme inducers is often gradual, and it can take up to 1 to 2 weeks for maximal effects, and from 1 to 4 weeks for the effect to dissipate (depending on which inducer is used).

OBJECT DRUGS	PRECIPITANT DRUGS
Antiarrhythmics	**Antidepressants**:
(CYP2D6 Substrates:	**Bupropion** (Wellbutrin)
Flecainide (Tambocor)	**Duloxetine** (Cymbalta)
Mexiletine (Mexitil)	**Fluoxetine** (Prozac)
Propafenone (Rythmol)	**Paroxetine** (Paxil)

COMMENTS: These antidepressants inhibit CYP2D6, and can lead to accumulation of flecainide, mexiletine, and propafenone, and increase the risk of toxicity. People with "normal" CYP2D6 activity (Extensive Metabolizers) are at the greatest risk.

CLASS 2: USE ONLY IF BENEFIT FELT TO OUTWEIGH RISK

- *Use Alternative*:

  Antidepressant: Citalopram (Celexa), **desvenlafaxine** (Pristiq), **escitalopram** (Lexapro), and **sertraline** (Zoloft), are weak inhibitors of CYP2D6, and **fluvoxamine** and **venlafaxine** (Effexor) have little or no effect on CYP2D6.

- *Monitor*: Be alert for an increased effect of the antiarrhythmic if CYP2D6 inhibitors are coadministered. Monitoring of the antiarrhythmic plasma concentration is warranted.

OBJECT DRUGS	PRECIPITANT DRUGS	
Antiarrhythmics	**Enzyme Inhibitors**	
(CYP2D6 Substrates:	**Amiodarone** (Cordarone)	**Propoxyphene** (Darvon)
Flecainide (Tambocor)	**Cinacalcet** (Sensipar)	**Quinidine** (Quinidex)
Mexiletine (Mexitil)	**Diphenhydramine** (Benadryl)	**Ritonavir** (Norvir)
Propafenone	**Haloperidol** (Haldol)	**Terbinafine** (Lamisil)
(Rythmol)	**Propafenone** (Rythmol)	**Thioridazine** (Mellaril)

COMMENTS: Drugs that inhibit CYP2D6 can lead to accumulation of flecainide, mexiletine, and propafenone, and increase the risk of toxicity. People with "normal" CYP2D6 activity (Extensive Metabolizers) are at the greatest risk. Note that because terbinafine has an extraordinarily long terminal half-life, the inhibitory effect of terbinafine on CYP2D6 may last for many weeks after terbinafine is discontinued.

CLASS 2: USE ONLY IF BENEFIT FELT TO OUTWEIGH RISK

- *Use Alternative*:
  Diphenhydramine: Other antihistamines such as **desloratadine** (Clarinex), **fexofenadine** (Allegra), **loratadine** Claritin), and **cetirizine** (Zyrtec) are not known to inhibit CYP2D6.
  Propoxyphene: Consider using an alternative analgesic; propoxyphene has limited efficacy, and other analgesics appear less likely to affect CYP2D6.
- *Monitor:* Be alert for an increased effect of the antiarrhythmic if CYP2D6 inhibitors are coadministered. Monitoring of the antiarrhythmic plasma concentration is warranted.

OBJECT DRUGS	PRECIPITANT DRUGS
Anticoagulants, Oral:	**Analgesics:**
Acenocoumarol	**Acetaminophen** (Tylenol)
Phenprocoumon	**Aspirin**
Warfarin (Coumadin)	

COMMENTS: Aspirin increases the risk of bleeding in anticoagulated patients due to inhibition of platelet function and gastric erosions. Large doses of aspirin (e.g. 3g/day or more) can increase the hypoprothrombinemic response. However, low (antiplatelet) doses of aspirin appear to increase primarily minor bleeding and the combination is used intentionally in many patients. Acetaminophen can increase the hypoprothrombinemic response to warfarin and probably other oral anticoagulants. In most cases the interaction is small, but in predisposed patients marked hypoprothrombinemia has been reported. It would be prudent to limit acetaminophen dosage to 2 g/day or less for no more than 4 or 5 days, and to monitor the INR.

CLASS 2: USE ONLY IF BENEFIT FELT TO OUTWEIGH RISK

- *Use Alternative:* As an analgesic, acetaminophen appears safer than aspirin for patients on warfarin (but avoid large or prolonged doses of acetaminophen). If a NSAID is required, see Anticoagulants, Oral + NSAIDs.
- *Circumvent/Minimize:* Advise patients on oral anticoagulants to avoid taking acetaminophen, aspirin or other salicylates unless instructed to do so by the prescriber of the oral anticoagulant.
- *Monitor:* Monitor the INR if acetaminophen or large doses of salicylates are given for more than a few days. Note that the increased bleeding risk from small doses of aspirin (e.g., less than 2 to 3 g/day) is usually not reflected in an increased INR or prothrombin time. Monitor carefully for clinical evidence of bleeding, especially from the gastrointestinal tract.

OBJECT DRUGS	PRECIPITANT DRUGS
Anticoagulants, Oral:	**Absorption Inhibitors:**
Acenocoumarol	**Cholestyramine** (Questran)
Phenprocoumon	**Colestipol** (Colestid)
Warfarin (Coumadin)	**Sucralfate** (Carafate)

COMMENTS: Bile acid binding resins and sucralfate bind with warfarin, phenprocoumon, and possibly other oral anticoagulants in the G.I. tract, thus reducing the anticoagulant absorption and response. Since warfarin and phenprocoumon undergo enterohepatic circulation, the binding cannot be completely avoided by spacing doses of the drugs.

CLASS 3: ASSESS RISK & TAKE ACTION IF NECESSARY

- *Circumvent/Minimize:* Give oral anticoagulants 2 hours before or 6 hours after absorption inhibitors; keep constant interval between doses of oral anticoagulant and absorption inhibitor.
- *Consider Alternative:* **Colesevelam** (Welchol) and **ezetimibe** (Zetia) do not appear to affect the bioavailability of warfarin.
- *Monitor:* Monitor response to anticoagulant if absorption inhibitor is initiated, discontinued, changed in dosage or if the interval between doses of the oral anticoagulant and the absorption inhibitor is changed.

OBJECT DRUGS	PRECIPITANT DRUGS	
Anticoagulants, Oral:	**Enzyme Inducers:**	
Acenocoumarol	**Azathioprine** (Imuran)	**Phenytoin** (Dilantin)
Phenprocoumon	**Barbiturates**	**Primidone** (Mysoline)
Warfarin (Coumadin)	**Carbamazepine** (Tegretol)	**Rifabutin** (Mycobutin)
	Dicloxacillin (Dynapen)	**Rifampin** (Rifadin)
	Griseofulvin (Grisactin)	**Rifapentine** (Priftin)
	Nafcillin (Unipen)	**St. John's Wort**
	Oxcarbazepine (Trileptal)	

COMMENTS: Enzyme inducers gradually reduce the anticoagulant response to oral anticoagulants. Phenytoin may actually *increase* warfarin effect initially—possibly by competitively inhibiting CYP2C9 activity and displacement of warfarin from plasma protein binding—but the initial increase is followed by reduced anticoagulant effect due to enzyme induction. Consider the increased risk of impaired anticoagulant control, and the increased monitoring cost, especially if the enzyme inducer will *not* be used chronically in a stable dose. Azathioprine appears to inhibit the anticoagulant effect of warfarin, but the mechanism for this effect is not clear. Theoretically, mercaptopurine may produce a similar effect on warfarin.

CLASS 2: USE ONLY IF BENEFIT FELT TO OUTWEIGH RISK

- *Use Alternative:*
  General: Suitable alternatives with equivalent efficacy are not available for most enzyme inducers. In patients stabilized on chronic therapy with the anticoagulant and an enzyme inducer, it may be better to maintain current

therapy, making sure the patient knows not to stop or change the dose of the enzyme inducer without consulting the prescriber of the anticoagulant.

St. John's Wort: Given the limited evidence of efficacy, St. John's Wort should generally be avoided in patients taking oral anticoagulants.

- **Monitor.** If it is necessary to use enzyme inducers and oral anticoagulants concurrently, monitor for altered response if the inducer is initiated, discontinued, or changed in dosage. Note that enzyme induction is often gradual; it can take up to 1 to 2 weeks or more for maximal effects, and from 1 to 4 weeks for the effect to dissipate (depending on which inducer is used).

OBJECT DRUGS	PRECIPITANT DRUGS
Anticoagulants, Oral:	**Enzyme Inhibitors:**
Acenocoumarol	**Alcohol** (intoxication)
Warfarin (Coumadin)	**Azapropazone**
	Sulfinpyrazone (Anturane)

COMMENTS: Acute alcohol intoxication can markedly increase the effect of warfarin. Azapropazon and sulfinpyrazone markedly increase the anticoagulant response to warfarin, due primarily to inhibition of CYP2C9 (assume that acenocoumarol interacts similarly until proved otherwise).

CLASS 1: AVOID COMBINATION

- **Avoid:** Patients receiving oral anticoagulants should avoid alcohol intoxication, but available evidence suggests that modest alcohol intake (e.g., 1-2 drinks/day) has little or no effect on warfarin response. Since azapropazone and sulfinpyrazone can markedly increase warfarin response, concurrent use should be avoided.

OBJECT DRUGS	PRECIPITANT DRUGS
Anticoagulants, Oral:	**HMG CoA Reductase Inhibitors:**
Acenocoumarol	**Fluvastatin** (Lescol)
Warfarin (Coumadin)	**Lovastatin** (Mevacor)
	Rosuvastatin (Crestor)
	Simvastatin (Zocor)

COMMENTS: Fluvastatin, and to a lesser degree, lovastatin and simvastatin, inhibit CYP2C9 and may increase the hypoprothrombinemic response to warfarin in some patients Rosuvastatin has been noted to increase the INR in patients taking warfarin.

CLASS 3: ASSESS RISK & TAKE ACTION IF NECESSARY

- **Consider Alternative:** Other HMG CoA reductase inhibitors such as **pravastatin** (Pravachol) and **atorvastatin** (Lipitor) appear to have little or no effect on warfarin response.
- **Monitor:** Monitor for altered warfarin response if fluvastatin, lovastatin, rosuvastatin, or simvastatin are initiated, discontinued, or changed in dosage.

OBJECT DRUGS	PRECIPITANT DRUGS
Anticoagulants, Oral:	**Azole Antifungals:**
Acenocoumarol	**Fluconazole** (Diflucan)
Warfarin (Coumadin)	**Miconazole** (Monistat)
	Voriconazole (Vfend)

COMMENTS: Fluconazole is a potent inhibitor of CYP2C9, and even at a dose of 100 mg/day can substantially increase the hypoprothrombinemic response of warfarin. Miconazole also strongly inhibits S-warfarin metabolism. Several cases have been reported of marked increase in warfarin effect following the use of miconazole oral gel, probably because the oral gel was swallowed and absorbed. Vaginal miconazole has also increased warfarin response in isolated cases. Topical administration of miconazole on the skin has been reported to increase warfarin effect, but the effect appears to be rare.

CLASS 2: USE ONLY IF BENEFIT FELT TO OUTWEIGH RISK

- *Use Alternative*: **Itraconazole** (Sporanox), **ketoconazole** (Nizoral), **posaconazole** (Noxafil), and **terbinafine** (Lamisil) probably have less effect on warfarin metabolism than other azole antifungals. Nonetheless, isolated cases of increased warfarin effect have been reported, and one should still monitor for increased warfarin response.
- *Monitor*: Monitor for altered hypoprothrombinemic response if an azole antifungal is initiated, discontinued, or changed in dosage.

OBJECT DRUGS	PRECIPITANT DRUGS
Anticoagulants, Oral:	**Cimetidine** (Tagamet)
Acenocoumarol	
Warfarin (Coumadin)	

COMMENTS: Cimetidine increases the hypoprothrombinemic response to warfarin. Although the effect is usually modest, it is also highly variable from patient to patient; hence, an occasional patient may develop a substantial increase in warfarin response.

CLASS 3: ASSESS RISK & TAKE ACTION IF NECESSARY

- *Consider Alternative*: Other acid suppressors are unlikely to interact. Consider using **famotidine** (Pepcid), **nizatidine** (Axid), **ranitidine** (Zantac), **deslansoprazole** (Kapidex), **lansoprazole** (Prevacid), **rabeprazole** (Aciphex), **omeprazole** (Prilosec), **esomeprazole** (Nexium), or **pantoprazole** (Protonix).
- *Monitor*: If the combination is used, monitor for altered warfarin response when cimetidine is initiated, discontinued, or changed in dosage.

OBJECT DRUGS	PRECIPITANT DRUGS
Anticoagulants, Oral:	**Antibiotics:**
Acenocoumarol	**Chloramphenicol** (Chloromycetin)
Warfarin (Coumadin)	**Co-trimoxazole** (Septra)
	Metronidazole (Flagyl)
	Sulfamethizole (Urobiotic)
	Sulfaphenazole

COMMENTS: Sulfamethoxazole (in co-trimoxazole) and metronidazole are known inhibitors of CYP2C9 and can substantially increase warfarin plasma concentrations and hypoprothrombinemic response. Chloramphenicol, also a CYP2C9 inhibitor, increases the hypoprothrombinemic response of dicumarol and probably also of warfarin. Many other antibiotics have been reported to increase warfarin response in isolated case reports, but these reports can be difficult to evaluate because such patients may have other risk factors for increased warfarin effect such as fever, poor oral intake, and acute illness. (See the Table **Effect of Other Antibiotics on Warfarin** at the end of the monographs.) Epidemiologic studies suggest that patients on warfarin who receive *any* antibiotic may be at increased risk for gastrointestinal bleeding.

CLASS 2: USE ONLY IF BENEFIT FELT TO OUTWEIGH RISK
- *Use Alternative:* Almost all antibiotics have been associated with increased warfarin response in at least a few patients, but most of them appear less likely to interact with warfarin than the antibiotics listed above.
- *Monitor:* If one of the antibiotics listed above must be used in a patient on warfarin, monitor anticoagulation carefully; an adjustment in warfarin dosage may be needed. Other antibiotics appear less likely to interact, but one should still monitor for altered effect.

OBJECT DRUGS	PRECIPITANT DRUGS
Anticoagulants, Oral:	**Antidepressants:**
Acenocoumarol	**Fluoxetine** (Prozac)
Warfarin (Coumadin)	**Fluvoxamine** (Luvox)

COMMENTS: CYP2C9 inhibitors increase S-warfarin concentrations; the onset of increased anticoagulant effect is usually gradual (over 7-10 days). Most studies involve warfarin, but assume that acenocoumarol interacts similarly until proved otherwise. Phenprocoumon is metabolized primarily by glucuronidation and theoretically would be unlikely to interact with CYP2C9 inhibitors.

CLASS 2: USE ONLY IF BENEFIT FELT TO OUTWEIGH RISK
- *Use Alternative:* Other SSRIs such as **citalopram** (Celexa), **escitalopram** (Lexapro), **desvenlafaxine** (Pristiq), **venlafaxine** (Effexor), **paroxetine** (Paxil) or **sertraline** (Zoloft) may be less likely to increase the hypoprothrombinemic response to warfarin, but SSRIs may increase bleeding risk even in the absence of increased INR response due to their antiplatelet effects.
- *Monitor:* Monitor for altered anticoagulant effect if fluvoxamine is initiated, discontinued, or changed in dosage.

OBJECT DRUGS	PRECIPITANT DRUGS	
Anticoagulants, Oral:	**Enzyme Inhibitors:**	
Acenocoumarol	**Amiodarone** (Cordarone)	**Imatinib** (Gleevec)
Warfarin (Coumadin)	**Androgens**	**Isoniazid** (INH)
	Capecitabine (Xeloda)	**Leflunomide** (Arava)
	Danazol (Danocrine)	**Mefloquine** (Lariam)
	Disulfiram (Antabuse)	**Propafenone** (Rythmol)
	Fenofibrate (Tricor)	**Tamoxifen** (Nolvadex)
	Fluorouracil (5-FU)	**Zafirlukast** (Accolate)
	Gemfibrozil (Lopid)	

COMMENTS: CYP2C9 inhibitors increase S-warfarin concentrations; the increased anticoagulant effect is usually gradual (over 7-10 days). The interaction magnitude varies considerably from patient to patient, and is usually dose related. Amiodarone may also increase oral anticoagulant response by increasing circulating thyroid hormone concentrations. The mechanism for the effect of androgens, danazol, and fibrates (clofibrate, fenofibrate, gemfibrozil) on warfarin response is not established. The leflunomide-warfarin interaction is based on limited clinical information. Most studies involve warfarin, but assume that acenocoumarol interacts similarly until proved otherwise. Phenprocoumon is primarily glucuronidated; it is unlikely to interact with CYP2C9 inhibitors.

CLASS 2: USE ONLY IF BENEFIT FELT TO OUTWEIGH RISK

- *Use Alternative*:
  Zafirlukast: **Montelukast** (Singulair) does not appear to interact with warfarin. **Zileuton** (Zyflo) may increase warfarin response somewhat, but probably to a lesser extent than zafirlukast.
- *Monitor*: If a CYP2C9 inhibitor is used, monitor for altered anticoagulant effect if inhibitor is initiated, discontinued, or changed in dosage. Amiodarone-induced inhibition may require several weeks to develop.

OBJECT DRUGS	PRECIPITANT DRUGS	
Anticoagulants, Oral:	**NSAIDs:**	
Acenocoumarol	**Diclofenac** (Voltaren)	**Meclofenamate**
Phenprocoumon	**Diflunisal** (Dolobid)	**Mefenamic acid**
Warfarin (Coumadin)	**Etodolac** (Lodine)	**Meloxicam** (Mobic)
	Fenoprofen (Nalfon)	**Nabumetone** (Relafen)
	Flurbiprofen (Ansaid)	**Naproxen** (Aleve)
	Ibuprofen (Motrin)	**Oxaprozin** (Daypro)
	Indomethacin (Indocin)	**Piroxicam** (Feldene)
	Ketoprofen (Orudis)	**Sulindac** (Clinoril)
	Ketorolac (Toradol)	**Tolmetin** (Tolectin)

COMMENTS: All NSAIDs reversibly inhibit platelet function and cause gastric erosions. The risk of GI bleeding appears to be considerably increased with NSAIDs plus warfarin compared to either drug used alone. Some NSAIDs can increase the hypoprothrombinemic response to oral anticoagulants.

CLASS 2: USE ONLY IF BENEFIT FELT TO OUTWEIGH RISK

- *Use Alternative*: Use a non-NSAID analgesic if possible such as acetaminophen (see Acetaminophen discussion under Anticoagulants, Oral + Aspirin). If a NSAID is required, non-acetylated salicylates such as choline magnesium trisalicylate (Trilisate), magnesium salicylates, and salsalate (Disalcid) are probably safer due to minimal effects on platelets and gastric mucosa; if large doses are used, monitor INR. COX-2 inhibitors produce no platelet inhibition and probably less gastric damage. Studies indicate that celecoxib does not affect warfarin response. However, isolated case reports of warfarin interactions with celecoxib have appeared, and epidemiologic evidence suggests that COX-2 inhibitors (celecoxib and rofexocib) may increase the risk of upper GI hemorrhage in patients on warfarin. If a standard NSAID is used, consider using NSAIDs that are unlikely to affect the hypoprothrombinemic response such as diclofenac (Voltaren), ibuprofen (Advil, Motrin), naproxen (Aleve), and tolmetin (Tolectin).
- *Monitor*: If any NSAID is used with an oral anticoagulant, monitor carefully for evidence of bleeding, especially from the GI tract.

OBJECT DRUGS	PRECIPITANT DRUGS
Anticoagulants, Oral:	**Thyroid:**
Acenocoumarol	Levothyroxine (Synthroid)
Phenprocoumon	Liothyronine (Cytomel)
Warfarin (Coumadin)	Liotrix (Thyrolar)
	Thyroid USP

COMMENTS: When thyroid hormones are started in the presence of oral anticoagulant therapy, the hypoprothrombinemic response increases gradually (thyroxine has a long half-life). The risk is probably minimal if anticoagulation therapy is started in a euthyroid patient stabilized on thyroid replacement therapy.

CLASS 3: ASSESS RISK & TAKE ACTION IF NECESSARY

- *Monitor*: Monitor for altered anticoagulant response if thyroid is initiated, discontinued or changed in dosage. Note that since the effect is gradual, monitoring may be needed for several weeks (sometimes more) until the hypoprothrombinemic response stabilizes.

OBJECT DRUGS	PRECIPITANT DRUGS	
Antidepressants, Tricyclic:	**Enzyme Inducers:**	
Amitriptyline (Elavil)	Barbiturates	Primidone (Mysoline)
Amoxapine (Asendin)	Carbamazepine (Tegretol)	Rifabutin
Clomipramine (Anafranil)	Efavirenz (Sustiva)	(Mycobutin)
Desipramine (Norpramin)	Nevirapine (Viramune)	Rifampin (Rifadin)
Doxepin (Sinequan)	Oxcarbazepine (Trileptal)	Rifapentine (Priftin)
Imipramine (Tofranil)	Phenytoin (Dilantin)	St. John's Wort
Nortriptyline (Aventyl)		
Protriptyline (Vivactil)		
Trimipramine (Surmontil)		

COMMENTS: Enzyme inducers may gradually reduce the serum levels and effect of imipramine, desipramine, amitriptyline, and probably other tricyclic antidepressants (TCA). TCAs differ in their metabolism by CYP450 isozymes; hence, the magnitude of TCAs interaction with enzyme inducers may vary as well.

CLASS 3: ASSESS RISK & TAKE ACTION IF NECESSARY

- *Consider Alternative*: While it would be prudent to use an alternative to the enzyme inducer, suitable alternatives with equivalent therapeutic effects are not available for most enzyme inducers. One could also consider a non-TCA antidepressant, but many of them may also be susceptible to enzyme induction.
- *Monitor*: Monitor for altered tricyclic antidepressant effect if enzyme inducer is initiated, discontinued, or changed in dosage. Keep in mind that enzyme induction is usually gradual and may take days to weeks for onset and offset, depending on the specific inducer.

OBJECT DRUGS	PRECIPITANT DRUGS
Antidepressants, Tricyclic:	**Antidepressants, Other:**
Amitriptyline (Elavil)	**Bupropion** (Wellbutrin)
Amoxapine (Asendin)	**Duloxetine** (Cymbalta)
Clomipramine (Anafranil)	**Fluoxetine** (Prozac)
Desipramine (Norpramin)	**Fluvoxamine** (Luvox)
Doxepin (Sinequan)	**Nefazodone**
Imipramine (Tofranil)	**Paroxetine** (Paxil)
Nortriptyline (Aventyl)	
Protriptyline (Vivactil)	
Trimipramine (Surmontil)	

COMMENTS: Antidepressants that inhibit CYP2D6 (and to a lesser extent inhibit CYP1A2 and CYP3A4) can increase tricyclic antidepressant (TCA) serum concentrations possibly leading to toxicity (e.g., dry mouth, urinary retention, blurred vision, tachycardia, constipation, and postural hypotension). With most inhibitors, the onset and offset of the interaction occurs over several days to a week, but it may take up to several weeks with fluoxetine. Combinations of TCAs and enzyme inhibitors (e.g., fluoxetine or paroxetine) are sometimes used intentionally to increase antidepressant efficacy.

CLASS 3: ASSESS RISK & TAKE ACTION IF NECESSARY

- *Consider Alternative*:
  Antidepressants, Other: **Sertraline** (Zoloft), **citalopram** (Celexa), **escitalopram** (Lexapro), **desvenlafaxine** (Pristiq), and **venlafaxine** (Effexor) have less effect on CYP2D6 than fluoxetine or paroxetine.
- *Monitor*: Monitor for altered TCA response if an SSRI that is an enzyme inhibitor is initiated, discontinued, or changed in dosage.

OBJECT DRUGS	PRECIPITANT DRUGS	
Antidepressants, Tricyclic:	**Enzyme Inhibitors:**	
Amitriptyline (Elavil)	**Amiodarone** (Cordarone)	**Propafenone**
Amoxapine (Asendin)	**Atazanavir** (Reyataz)	(Rythmol)
Clomipramine (Anafranil)	**Cimetidine** (Tagamet)	**Propoxyphene**
Desipramine (Norpramin)	**Cinacalcet** (Sensipar)	(Darvon)
Doxepin (Sinequan)	**Conivaptan** (Vaprisol)	**Quinidine** (Quinidex)
Imipramine (Tofranil)	**Diphenhydramine**	**Ranolazine** (Ranexa)
Nortriptyline (Aventyl)	(Benadryl)	**Ritonavir** (Norvir)
Protriptyline (Vivactil)	**Haloperidol** (Haldol)	**Terbinafine** (Lamisil)
Trimipramine (Surmontil)		**Thioridazine**
		(Mellaril)

COMMENTS: CYP2D6 inhibitors (and to a lesser extent inhibitors of CYP1A2 and CYP3A4) can increase tricyclic antidepressant (TCA) serum concentrations possibly leading to toxicity (e.g., dry mouth, urinary retention, blurred vision, tachycardia, constipation, and postural hypotension). Both bupropion and tricyclic antidepressants can lower the seizure threshold, so theoretically the combination may increase the risk of seizures. Note that because terbinafine has an extraordinarily long terminal half-life, the inhibitory effect of terbinafine on CYP2D6 may last for many weeks after terbinafine is discontinued.

CLASS 3: ASSESS RISK & TAKE ACTION IF NECESSARY

- *Consider Alternative*:
  Cimetidine: Other acid suppressors are unlikely to interact. Consider using **famotidine** (Pepcid), **nizatidine** (Axid), **ranitidine** (Zantac), **deslansoprazole** (Kapidex), **esomeprazole** (Nexium), **omeprazole** (Prilosec), **lansoprazole** (Prevacid), **rabeprazole** (Aciphex), or **pantoprazole** (Protonix).
  Diphenhydramine: Nonsedating antihistamines are unlikely to inhibit CYP2D6.
- *Monitor*: Monitor for altered TCA response if an enzyme inhibitor is initiated, discontinued, or changed in dosage.

OBJECT DRUGS	PRECIPITANT DRUGS
Antidiabetic Agents:	**Beta-Blockers, Nonselective:**
Chlorpropamide (Diabinese)	**Carteolol** (Ocupress)
Glimepiride (Amaryl)	**Carvedilol** (Coreg)
Glipizide (Glucotrol)	**Labetalol** (Trandate)
Glyburide (DiaBeta, Glucovance)	**Nadolol** (Corgard)
Insulin	**Penbutolol** (Levatol)
Metformin (Glucophage)	**Pindolol** (Visken)
Nateglinide (Starlix)	**Propranolol** (Inderal)
Pioglitazone (Actos)	**Sotalol** (Betapace)
Repaglinide (Prandin)	**Timolol** (Blocadren)
Rosiglitazone (Avandia)	
Saxagliptin (Onglyza)	
Tolbutamide (Orinase)	

COMMENTS: Noncardioselective beta-adrenergic blockers may prolong the duration of a hypoglycemic reaction; patients may also develop hypertensive reactions with compensatory bradycardia during hypoglycemia. All beta-blockers inhibit hypoglycemia-induced tachycardia, but sweating is not inhibited.

CLASS 2: USE ONLY IF BENEFIT FELT TO OUTWEIGH RISK

- *Use Alternative:* Avoid nonselective beta-adrenergic blockers in patients receiving antidiabetic agents if possible. If beta-blockers are used, cardioselective agents are preferred, since they are less likely to prolong hypoglycemia or produce hypertensive reactions during hypoglycemia. Cardioselective beta-blockers include **acebutolol** (Sectral), **atenolol** (Tenormin), **betaxolol** (Kerlone), **bisoprolol** (Zebeta) and **metoprolol** (Lopressor).
- *Monitor:* Diabetic patients taking beta-blockers should be warned that hypoglycemic episodes may not result in tachycardia.

OBJECT DRUGS	PRECIPITANT DRUGS
Antidiabetic Agents	**Azole Antifungals:**
(CYP2C9 Substrates):	**Fluconazole** (Diflucan)
Chlorpropamide (Diabinese)	**Voriconazole** (Vfend)
Glimepiride (Amaryl)	
Glipizide (Glucotrol)	
Glyburide (DiaBeta)	
Nateglinide (Starlix)	
Rosiglitazone (Avandia)	
Tolbutamide (Orinase)	

COMMENTS: Oral hypoglycemic drugs that are metabolized by CYP2C9 may produce enhanced hypoglycemic effects when administered with azole antifungal agents that inhibit the enzyme. Nateglinide and rosiglitazone both have additional pathways of metabolism and may be less affected by inhibitors of only one pathway.

CLASS 3: ASSESS RISK & TAKE ACTION IF NECESSARY

- *Consider Alternative:* Itraconazole (Sporanox) and **terbinafine** (Lamisil) are antifungals that do not inhibit CYP2C9. **Ketoconazole** (Nizoral) has been reported to increase the plasma concentrations of rosiglitazone and tolbutamide.
- *Monitor:* Diabetic patients taking CYP2C9-inhibiting antifungals should be warned that hypoglycemic episodes may occur more frequently and should monitor their blood glucose concentrations.

OBJECT DRUGS	PRECIPITANT DRUGS
Antidiabetic Agents:	**Enzyme Inhibitors:**
(CYP2C9 Substrates):	**Amiodarone** (Cordarone)
Chlorpropamide (Diabinese)	**Capecitabine** (Xeloda)
Glimepiride (Amaryl)	**Co-trimoxazole** (Septra)
Glipizide (Glucotrol)	**Delavirdine** (Rescriptor)
Glyburide (DiaBeta, Glucovance)	**Efavirenz** (Sustiva)
Nateglinide (Starlix)	**Fluorouracil** (5-FU)
Rosiglitazone (Avandia)	**Fluoxetine** (Prozac)
Tolbutamide (Orinase)	**Fluvastatin** (Lescol)
	Fluvoxamine (Luvox)
	Metronidazole (Flagyl)
	Sulfinpyrazone (Anturane)

COMMENTS: Oral hypoglycemic drugs that are metabolized by CYP2C9 may produce enhanced hypoglycemic effects when administered with a CYP2C9 inhibitor. Nateglinide and rosiglitazone both have additional pathways of metabolism and may be less affected by inhibitors of only one pathway. Co-trimoxazole, however, inhibits two pathways for rosiglitazone metabolism; the trimethoprim component inhibits CYP2C8, and the sulfamethoxazole component inhibits CYP2C9. Single doses of metronidazole would be unlikely to produce hypoglycemia when combined with these antidiabetic agents.

CLASS 3: ASSESS RISK & TAKE ACTION IF NECESSARY
- *Consider Alternative*:
  Fluvastatin: **Atorvastatin** (Lipitor), **lovastatin** (Mevacor), **pravastatin** (Pravachol), **rosuvastatin** (Crestor), and **simvastatin** (Zocor) do not appear to inhibit CYP2C9.
  Fluoxetine / Fluvoxamine: Other SSRI antidepressants would not be expected to interact.
- *Monitor*: Monitor for hypoglycemic episodes during coadministration of CYP2C9 inhibitors.

OBJECT DRUGS	PRECIPITANT DRUGS	
Antidiabetic Agents	**Antimicrobials:**	
(CYP3A4 Substrates):	**Clarithromycin** (Biaxin)	**Posaconazole** (Noxafil)
Nateglinide (Starlix)	**Erythromycin** (E-Mycin)	**Quinupristin** (Synercid)
Pioglitazone (Actos)	**Fluconazole** (Diflucan)	**Telithromycin** (Ketek)
Repaglinide (Prandin)	**Isoniazid** (INH)	**Troleandomycin** (TAO)
Saxagliptin (Onglyza)	**Itraconazole** (Sporanox)	**Voriconazole** (Vfend)
	Ketoconazole (Nizoral)	

COMMENTS: Some antimicrobials can reduce oral hypoglycemic metabolism and produce hypoglycemic episodes. Pioglitazone and repaglinide are also metabolized by CYP2C8, and people taking a CYP2C8 inhibitor in addition to a CYP3A4 inhibitor may have large interactions. For example, patients taking repaglinide with both gemfibrozil (CYP2C8 inhibitor) and itraconazole (CYP3A4 inhibitor) may have 20-fold increases in repaglinide plasma concentrations. (See CYP Table at front of book for other CYP2C8 inhibitors.)

CLASS 3: ASSESS RISK & TAKE ACTION IF NECESSARY
- *Consider Alternative*:
  Azole Antifungals: Fluconazole appears to be a less potent inhibitor of CYP3A4; but in larger doses it also inhibits CYP3A4. **Terbinafine** (Lamisil) does not appear to affect CYP3A4.
  Macrolide Antibiotics: **Azithromycin** (Zithromax) and **dirithromycin*** do not appear to inhibit CYP3A4 and are unlikely to interact. (*not available in US)
  Telithromycin: The use of **azithromycin** (Zithromax) or a quinolone antibiotic should be considered.
  Saxagliptin: Another DPP-4 inhibitor, **sitagliptin** (Januvia) is largely excreted unchanged in the urine; theoretically, it would be unlikely to interact with CYP3A4 inhibitors.
- *Monitor*: Monitor for hypoglycemic episodes during azole antifungal or macrolide coadministration.

OBJECT DRUGS	PRECIPITANT DRUGS
Antidiabetic Agents (CYP3A4 Substrates):	**Calcium Channel Blockers**
Nateglinide (Starlix)	**Diltiazem** (Cardizem)
Pioglitazone (Actos)	**Verapamil** (Isoptin)
Repaglinide (Prandin)	
Saxagliptin (Onglyza)	

COMMENTS: Diltiazem and verapamil (both are CYP3A4 inhibitors) could reduce oral hypoglycemic metabolism and produce hypoglycemic episodes. Pioglitazone and repaglinide are also metabolized by CYP2C8, and people taking a CYP2C8 inhibitor in addition to a CYP3A4 inhibitor may have large interactions. For example, patients taking repaglinide with both gemfibrozil (CYP2C8 inhibitor) and itraconazole (CYP3A4 inhibitor may have 20-fold increases in repaglinide plasma concentrations. (See CYP Table at front of book for other CYP2C8 inhibitors.)

CLASS 3: ASSESS RISK & TAKE ACTION IF NECESSARY
- *Consider Alternative*:
  Calcium channel blockers: Agents other than diltiazem and verapamil are unlikely to inhibit the metabolism of these antidiabetic agents.
  Saxagliptin: Another DPP-4 inhibitor, **sitagliptin** (Januvia) is largely excreted unchanged in the urine; theoretically, it would be unlikely to interact with CYP3A4 inhibitors.
- *Monitor*: Monitor for hypoglycemic episodes during calcium channel blocker coadministration.

OBJECT DRUGS	PRECIPITANT DRUGS	
Antidiabetic Agents	**Enzyme Inhibitors:**	
CYP3A4 Substrates):	**Amiodarone** (Cordarone)	**Fluvoxamine** (Luvox)
Nateglinide (Starlix)	**Amprenavir** (Agenerase)	**Grapefruit**
Pioglitazone (Actos)	**Aprepitant** (Emend)	**Indinavir** (Crixivan)
Repaglinide (Prandin)	**Atazanavir** (Reyataz)	**Nefazodone**
Saxagliptin (Onglyza)	**Conivaptan** (Vaprisol)	**Nelfinavir** (Viracept)
	Cyclosporine (Neoral)	**Ritonavir** (Norvir)
	Darunavir (Prezista)	**Saquinavir** (Invirase)
	Delavirdine (Rescriptor)	

COMMENTS: Although data are limited, any CYP3A4 inhibitor could reduce oral hypoglycemic metabolism and produce hypoglycemic episodes. Pioglitazone and repaglinide are also metabolized by CYP2C8, and people taking a CYP2C8 inhibitor in addition to a CYP3A4 inhibitor may have large interactions. For example, patients taking repaglinide with both gemfibrozil (CYP2C8 inhibitor) and itraconazole (CYP3A4 inhibitor may have 20-fold increases in repaglinide plasma concentrations. (See CYP Table at front of book for other CYP2C8 inhibitors.)

CLASS 3: ASSESS RISK & TAKE ACTION IF NECESSARY
- *Consider Alternative*:
  Antidepressants: Sertraline (Zoloft), citalopram (Celexa), escitalopram (Lexapro), desvenlafaxine (Pristiq), venlafaxine (Effexor), and paroxetine (Paxil) appear less likely to inhibit CYP3A4 than fluvoxamine. Fluoxetine (Prozac) appears to be a weak inhibitor of CYP3A4.
  Grapefruit: Orange juice does not appear to inhibit CYP3A4.
  Saxagliptin: Another DPP-4 inhibitor, sitagliptin (Januvia) is largely excreted unchanged in the urine; theoretically, it would be unlikely to interact with CYP3A4 inhibitors.
- *Monitor:* Monitor for hypoglycemic episodes during the coadministration of CYP3A4 inhibitors.

OBJECT DRUGS	PRECIPITANT DRUGS	
Antidiabetic Agents:	**Gastric Alkalinizers:**	
Glipizide (Glucotrol)	**Antacids**	**Lansoprazole** (Prevacid)
Glyburide (DiaBeta,	**Cimetidine** (Tagamet)	**Nizatidine** (Axid)
Glucovance)	**Deslansoprazole**	**Omeprazole** (Prilosec)
	(Kapidex)	**Pantoprazole** (Protonix)
	Esomeprazole (Nexium)	**Rabeprazole** (Aciphex)
	Famotidine (Pepcid)	**Ranitidine** (Zantac)

COMMENTS: Antacids have been reported to increase the rate or amount of absorption of glipizide and glyburide and to increase their hypoglycemic effects. Ranitidine was reported to increase the hypoglycemic effects of glipizide. If these effects are due to changes in gastric pH, other gastric alkalinizers would likely have a similar effect.

CLASS 3: ASSESS RISK & TAKE ACTION IF NECESSARY

- **Circumvent/Minimize:** Administration of the glipizide or glyburide two hours before an antacid would avoid the interactions. It may be difficult to separate the doses of an H$_2$-antagonist or PPI to ensure no interaction occurs.
- **Consider Alternative:** Other oral hypoglycemic agents such as **chlorpropamide** (Diabinese), **metformin** (Glucophage), **tolbutamide** (Orinase), or **rosiglitazone** (Avandia) may avoid interactions with gastric alkalinizers.
- **Monitor:** The administration of gastric alkalinizers to patients taking glipizide or glyburide should be accompanied by careful blood glucose monitoring.

OBJECT DRUGS	PRECIPITANT DRUGS	
Antihypertensive Drugs:	**NSAIDs:**	
ACE Inhibitors (ACEIs)	**Aspirin**	**Meclofenamate**
Angiotensin Receptor	**Diclofenac** (Voltaren)	**Mefenamic acid**
Blockers (ARBs)	**Diflunisal** (Dolobid)	**Meloxicam** (Mobic)
	Etodolac (Lodine)	**Nabumetone** (Relafen)
	Fenoprofen (Nalfon)	**Naproxen** (Aleve)
	Flurbiprofen (Ansaid)	**Oxaprozin** (Daypro)
	Ibuprofen (Motrin)	**Piroxicam** (Feldene)
	Indomethacin (Indocin)	**Sulindac** (Clinoril)
	Ketoprofen (Orudis)	**Tolmetin** (Tolectin)
	Ketorolac (Toradol)	

COMMENTS: In patients receiving ACEIs or ARBs for hypertension concurrent use of NSAIDs can substantially reduce the antihypertensive response. In most cases the effect is gradual, so short-term use of NSAIDs (i.e., a few days) in patients with well-controlled hypertension is unlikely to cause problems. Low-dose aspirin does not appear to have much effect on antihypertensive therapy. NSAIDs may also interfere with the efficacy of ACEIs, ARBs and diuretics used in the treatment of heart failure.

CLASS 3: ASSESS RISK & TAKE ACTION IF NECESSARY

- **Consider Alternative:**

NSAID: If possible use a non-NSAID analgesic such as acetaminophen. If a NSAID is required, use the lowest effective dose. There is some evidence to suggest that certain NSAIDs may have less effect than others on blood pressure, so if one NSAID is a problem, consider trying a different NSAID. It is not established that COX-2 inhibitors such as **celecoxib** (Celebrex) avoid the interaction but they could be tried. Because non-acetylated salicylates such as **choline magnesium trisalicylate** (Trilisate), **magnesium salicylates**, and **salsalate** (Disalcid) have less effect on prostaglandins than aspirin, they may be less likely to interact.

Antihypertensive: Although ACEIs and ARBs appear to be particularly susceptible to interactions with NSAIDs, diuretics and other antihypertensives may be affected as well. Nonetheless, in cases where it is not possible to modify the NSAID therapy, it may be possible to control the hypertension by using antihypertensive agents other than ACEIs or ARBs. Some recommend the use of calcium channel blockers if NSAIDs are preventing antihypertensive control.

- **_Monitor_:** If NSAIDs are used in patients on antihypertensive therapy, monitor the blood pressure carefully. Keep in mind that the effect may take place gradually over 2 to 3 weeks after starting the NSAID. Blood pressure monitoring is also warranted if the NSAID dose is changed or discontinued, or if the patient is switched from one NSAID to another.

OBJECT DRUGS	PRECIPITANT DRUGS
Antimetabolites:	**Allopurinol** (Zyloprim)
Azathioprine (Imuran)	**Febuxostat** (Uloric)
Mercaptopurine (Purinethol)	

COMMENTS: Allopurinol and febuxostat inhibit the metabolism of mercaptopurine, which is also the active metabolite of azathioprine. This effect considerably increases antimetabolite effect and toxicity of both azathioprine and mercaptopurine. Generally, these combinations should be avoided, but they have sometimes been used intentionally with careful monitoring.

CLASS 1: AVOID COMBINATION
- **_Avoid_:** Patients taking azathioprine or mercaptopurine should generally not be administered allopurinol or febuxostat. If allopurinol or febuxostat must be used, consider selecting an alternative immunosuppressant.

OBJECT DRUGS		PRECIPITANT DRUGS
Anxiolytics		**Antidepressants:**
(CYP3A4 substrates):		**Fluvoxamine** (Luvox)
Alprazolam (Xanax)	**Flurazepam** (Dalmane)	**Nefazodone**
Buspirone (BuSpar)	**Halazepam** (Paxipam)	
Clonazepam (Klonopin)	**Midazolam** (Versed), oral	
Clorazepate (Tranxene)	**Prazepam** (Centrex)	
Diazepam (Valium)	**Triazolam** (Halcion)	
Estazolam (ProSom)		

COMMENTS: When given orally, alprazolam, midazolam and triazolam undergo extensive first pass metabolism by CYP3A4 in the gut wall and liver. Other benzodiazepines such as clonazepam, clorazepate, diazepam, flurazepam, halazepam, and prazepam are also at least partly metabolized by CYP3A4, and may also interact with CYP3A4 inhibitors. Intravenous midazolam is less affected than when it is given orally. The primary risk of these interactions is impairment of motor skills that could result in falls or motor vehicle accidents.

CLASS 3: ASSESS RISK & TAKE ACTION IF NECESSARY
- **_Consider Alternative_:**
  Benzodiazepines: Consider other benzodiazepines: **temazepam** (Restoril), **oxazepam** (Serax), and **lorazepam** (Ativan) are largely glucuronidated, and are unlikely to be affected by CYP3A4 inhibitors.
  Antidepressants: **Sertraline** (Zoloft), **citalopram** (Celexa), **escitalopram** (Lexapro), **desvenlafaxine** (Pristiq), **venlafaxine** (Effexor), **paroxetine** (Paxil),

and **duloxetine** (Cymbalta) appear less likely to inhibit CYP3A4 than fluvoxamine or nefazodone.

- *Monitor*: Monitor for altered benzodiazepine response if the CYP3A4 inhibitor is initiated, discontinued, or changed in dosage. Warn patients about increased sedative effects.

OBJECT DRUGS	PRECIPITANT DRUGS
Anxiolytics (CYP3A4 Substrates):	**Antimicrobials:**
Alprazolam (Xanax)	**Clarithromycin** (Biaxin)
Buspirone (BuSpar)	**Erythromycin** (E-Mycin)
Clonazepam (Klonopin)	**Fluconazole** (Diflucan)
Clorazepate (Tranxene)	**Itraconazole** (Sporanox)
Diazepam (Valium)	**Ketoconazole** (Nizoral)
Estazolam (ProSom)	**Posaconazole** (Noxafil)
Flurazepam (Dalmane)	**Quinupristin** (Synercid)
Halazepam (Paxipam)	**Telithromycin** (Ketek)
Midazolam (Versed), oral	**Troleandomycin** (TAO)
Prazepam (Centrex)	**Voriconazole** (Vfend)
Triazolam (Halcion)	

COMMENTS: When given orally, alprazolam, midazolam and triazolam undergo extensive first pass metabolism by CYP3A4 in the gut wall and liver, so CYP3A4 inhibitors can dramatically increase plasma concentrations. Other benzodiazepines such as clonazepam, clorazepate, diazepam, flurazepam, halazepam, and prazepam are also partly metabolized by CYP3A4. Intravenous midazolam is much less affected than oral midazolam. The primary risk of these interactions is impairment of motor skills that could result in falls or motor vehicle accidents.

CLASS 3: ASSESS RISK & TAKE ACTION IF NECESSARY
- *Consider Alternative*:
  Azole Antifungals: Fluconazole appears to be a less potent inhibitor of CYP3A4; but in larger doses it also inhibits CYP3A4. **Terbinafine** (Lamisil) does not appear to affect CYP3A4.
  Benzodiazepines: Consider other benzodiazepines: **temazepam** (Restoril), **oxazepam** (Serax), and **lorazepam** (Ativan) are largely glucuronidated, and unlikely to be affected by CYP3A4 inhibitors.
  Macrolide Antibiotics: Unlike erythromycin, clarithromycin and troleandomycin, **azithromycin** (Zithromax) and **dirithromycin*** do not appear to inhibit CYP3A4. (*not available in US)
  Telithromycin: The use of **azithromycin** (Zithromax) or a quinolone antibiotic should be considered.
- *Monitor*: Monitor for altered benzodiazepine response if CYP3A4 inhibitor is initiated, discontinued or changed in dose. Warn patients about increased sedative effects.

OBJECT DRUGS	PRECIPITANT DRUGS
Anxiolytics	**Calcium Channel Blockers:**
(CYP3A4 substrates):	**Diltiazem** (Cardizem)
Alprazolam (Xanax)	**Verapamil** (Isoptin)
Buspirone (BuSpar)	
Clonazepam (Klonopin)	
Clorazepate (Tranxene)	
Diazepam (Valium)	
Estazolam (ProSom)	
Flurazepam (Dalmane)	
Halazepam (Paxipam)	
Midazolam (Versed), oral	
Prazepam (Centrex)	
Triazolam (Halcion)	

COMMENTS: When given orally, alprazolam, midazolam and triazolam undergo extensive first pass metabolism by CYP3A4 in the gut wall and liver. Other benzodiazepines such as clonazepam, clorazepate, diazepam, flurazepam, halazepam, and prazepam are also at least partly metabolized by CYP3A4, and may also interact with CYP3A4 inhibitors, Intravenous midazolam is much less affected than when it is given orally. The primary risk of these interactions is impairment of motor skills that could result in falls or motor vehicle accidents.

CLASS 3: ASSESS RISK & TAKE ACTION IF NECESSARY

- *Consider Alternative*:
  Benzodiazepines: Consider other benzodiazepines: **temazepam** (Restoril), **oxazepam** (Serax), and **lorazepam** (Ativan) are largely glucuronidated, and are unlikely to be affected by CYP3A4 inhibitors.
  Calcium Channel Blockers: Calcium channel blockers other than diltiazem and verapamil are unlikely to inhibit the metabolism of benzodiazepines.
- *Monitor*: Monitor for altered benzodiazepine response if the CYP3A4 inhibitor is initiated, discontinued, or changed in dosage. Warn patients about increased sedative effects.

OBJECT DRUGS	PRECIPITANT DRUGS
Anxiolytics (CYP3A4 substrates):	**Enzyme Inhibitors:**
Alprazolam (Xanax)	**Amiodarone** (Cordarone)
Buspirone (BuSpar)	**Amprenavir** (Agenerase)
Clonazepam (Klonopin)	**Aprepitant** (Emend)
Clorazepate (Tranxene)	**Atazanavir** (Reyataz)
Diazepam (Valium)	**Conivaptan** (Vaprisol)
Estazolam (ProSom)	**Cyclosporine** (Neoral)
Flurazepam (Dalmane)	**Darunavir** (Prezista)
Halazepam (Paxipam)	**Delavirdine** (Rescriptor)
Midazolam (Versed), oral	**Grapefruit**
Prazepam (Centrex)	**Indinavir** (Crixivan)
Triazolam (Halcion)	**Nelfinavir** (Viracept)
	Ritonavir (Norvir)
	Saquinavir (Invirase)

COMMENTS: When given orally, alprazolam, midazolam and triazolam, undergo extensive first pass metabolism by CYP3A4 in the gut wall and liver. Other benzodiazepines such as clonazepam, clorazepate, diazepam, flurazepam, halazepam, and prazepam are also at least partly metabolized by CYP3A4, and may also interact with CYP3A4 inhibitors. Intravenous midazolam is less affected than when it is given orally. The primary risk of these interactions is impairment of motor skills that could result in falls or motor vehicle accidents. Some of these combinations are listed as contraindicated by the manufacturer (e.g., amprenavir and atazanavir with midazolam or triazolam).

CLASS 3: ASSESS RISK & TAKE ACTION IF NECESSARY
- *Consider Alternative*:
  Benzodiazepines: Consider other benzodiazepines: **temazepam** (Restoril), **oxazepam** (Serax), and **lorazepam** (Ativan) arc largely glucuronidated, and are unlikely to be affected by CYP3A4 inhibitors.
  Grapefruit: Orange juice does not appear to inhibit CYP3A4.
- *Monitor*: Monitor for altered benzodiazepine response if the CYP3A4 inhibitor is initiated, discontinued, or changed in dosage. Warn patients about increased sedative effects.

OBJECT DRUGS	PRECIPITANT DRUGS	
Aripiprazole (Abilify)	**Enzyme Inducers:**	
	Barbiturates	**Phenytoin** (Dilantin)
	Bosentan (Tracleer)	**Primidone** (Mysoline)
	Carbamazepine	**Rifabutin** (Mycobutin)
	(Tegretol)	**Rifampin** (Rifadin)
	Efavirenz (Sustiva)	**Rifapentine** (Priftin)
	Nevirapine (Viramune)	**St. John's Wort**
	Oxcarbazepine (Trileptal)	

COMMENTS: Aripiprazole is metabolized by CYP3A4 and CYP2D6; drugs that induce CYP3A4 may reduce the serum levels of aripiprazole resulting in loss of efficacy. (CYP2D6 is not as susceptible to enzyme induction.)

CLASS 3: ASSESS RISK & TAKE ACTION IF NECESSARY
- *Consider Alternative:* Use an alternative to the enzyme inducer if possible.
- *Circumvent/Minimize:* The manufacturer recommends that the dose of aripiprazole be doubled (to 20-30 mg/day) if CYP3A4 inducers are added. If the enzyme inducer is then discontinued, they recommend that the aripiprazole dose be decreased to 10-15 mg/day.
- *Monitor:* If it is necessary to use aripiprazole and enzyme inducers monitor for altered aripiprazole effect if an enzyme inducer is started, stopped, or changed in dosage. Keep in mind that enzyme induction is usually gradual and may take days to weeks for onset and offset, depending on the specific inducer.

OBJECT DRUGS	PRECIPITANT DRUGS
Aripiprazole (Abilify)	<u>**Antimicrobials:**</u>
	Clarithromycin (Biaxin)
	Erythromycin (E-Mycin)
	Fluconazole (Diflucan)
	Itraconazole (Sporanox)
	Ketoconazole (Nizoral)
	Posaconazole (Noxafil)
	Quinupristin (Synercid)
	Telithromycin (Ketek)
	Troleandomycin (TAO)
	Voriconazole (Vfend)

COMMENTS: Aripiprazole is metabolized by CYP3A4 and CYP2D6; these antimicrobials inhibit CYP3A4, and may increase aripiprazole serum levels. Theoretically, patients with genetically reduced CYP2D6 activity or who are taking CYP2D6 inhibitors would be at greater risk from these interactions.

CLASS 3: ASSESS RISK & TAKE ACTION IF NECESSARY
- *Consider Alternative:*
  Azole Antifungals: Itraconazole and ketoconazole are potent inhibitors of CYP3A4; fluconazole appears weaker, but in larger doses it also inhibits CYP3A4. **Terbinafine** (Lamisil) does not appear to affect CYP3A4, but it does inhibit CYP2D6; thus, it would be expected to interact with aripiprazole.
  Macrolide Antibiotics: Unlike erythromycin, clarithromycin and troleandomycin, **azithromycin** (Zithromax) and **dirithromycin*** do not appear to inhibit CYP3A4. (*not available in US)
  Telithromycin: The use of **azithromycin** (Zithromax) or a quinolone antibiotic may be considered.
- *Circumvent/Minimize:* The manufacturer recommends that the dose of aripiprazole be reduced to one-half the usual dose if CYP3A4 inhibitors are added. If the CYP3A4 inhibitor is then discontinued, they recommend that the aripiprazole dose be increased to the usual dosage.

- *Monitor*: Be alert for altered effect of aripiprazole if CYP2D6 inhibitors are started, stopped, or changed in dosage. Due to the long half-life of aripiprazole and its active metabolite, the onset and offset of these interactions may take one to two weeks.

OBJECT DRUGS	PRECIPITANT DRUGS
Aripiprazole (Abilify)	<u>Antidepressants:</u> **Bupropion** (Wellbutrin) **Duloxetine** (Cymbalta) **Fluoxetine** (Prozac) **Fluvoxamine** (Luvox) **Nefazodone** **Paroxetine** (Paxil)

COMMENTS: Aripiprazole is metabolized by CYP2D6 and CYP3A4. These antidepressants inhibit either CYP2D6 or CYP3A4, and may lead to accumulation of aripiprazole.

CLASS 3: ASSESS RISK & TAKE ACTION IF NECESSARY

- *Consider Alternative*: Antidepressants with small or no effects on either CYP3A4 or CYP2D6 include **citalopram** (Celexa), **escitalopram** (Lexapro), **venlafaxine** (Effexor), **desvenlafaxine** (Pristiq), and **sertraline** (Zoloft),
- *Circumvent/Minimize*: The manufacturer recommends that the dose of aripiprazole be reduced to one-half the usual dose if CYP2D6 inhibitors or CYP3A4 inhibitors are added. If the inhibitor is then discontinued, they recommend that the aripiprazole dose be increased to the usual dosage.
- *Monitor*: Be alert for altered effect of aripiprazole if CYP2D6 inhibitors or CYP3A4 inhibitors are started, stopped, or changed in dosage. Due to the long half-life of aripiprazole and its active metabolite, the onset and offset of these interactions may take one to two weeks.

OBJECT DRUGS	PRECIPITANT DRUGS	
Aripiprazole (Abilify)	<u>Enzyme Inhibitors:</u> <u>(CYP3A4)</u> **Amiodarone** (Cordarone) **Amprenavir** (Agenerase) **Aprepitant** (Emend) **Atazanavir** (Reyataz) **Conivaptan** (Vaprisol) **Cyclosporine** (Neoral) **Darunavir** (Prezista) **Delavirdine** (Rescriptor)	 **Diltiazem** (Cardizem) **Grapefruit** **Indinavir** (Crixivan) **Nelfinavir** (Viracept) **Ritonavir** (Norvir) **Saquinavir** (Invirase) **Verapamil** (Isoptin)

COMMENTS: Aripiprazole is metabolized by CYP3A4 and CYP2D6; these drugs inhibit CYP3A4, and may increase aripiprazole serum levels. Theoretically, patients with genetically reduced CYP2D6 activity or who are taking CYP2D6 inhibitors would be at greater risk from these interactions.

CLASS 3: ASSESS RISK & TAKE ACTION IF NECESSARY

- *Consider Alternative:* Use an alternative to the enzyme inhibitor if possible.
  <u>Calcium channel blockers</u>: Calcium channel blockers other than diltiazem and verapamil are unlikely to inhibit CYP3A4.
  <u>Grapefruit</u>: Orange juice does not appear to inhibit CYP3A4.
- *Circumvent/Minimize:* The manufacturer recommends that the dose of aripiprazole be reduced to one-half the usual dose if CYP3A4 inhibitors or CYP2D6 inhibitors are added. If the inhibitor is then discontinued, they recommend that the aripiprazole dose be increased to the usual dosage.
- *Monitor:* Be alert for altered effect of aripiprazole if CYP3A4 inhibitors are started, stopped, or changed in dosage.

OBJECT DRUGS	PRECIPITANT DRUGS	
Aripiprazole (Abilify)	<u>**Enzyme Inhibitors:**</u> <u>**(CYP2D6)**</u>	
	Amiodarone (Cordarone)	**Propoxyphene** (Darvon)
	Cinacalcet (Sensipar)	**Quinidine** (Quinidex)
	Diphenhydramine (Benadryl)	**Ritonavir** (Norvir)
	Haloperidol (Haldol)	**Terbinafine** (Lamisil)
	Propafenone (Rythmol)	**Thioridazine** (Mellaril)

COMMENTS: Aripiprazole is metabolized by CYP2D6 and CYP3A4. These drugs inhibit CYP2D6, and may lead to accumulation of aripiprazole. People with "normal" CYP2D6 activity (Extensive Metabolizers) are at the greatest risk. Note that because terbinafine has an extraordinarily long terminal half-life, the inhibitory effect of terbinafine on CYP2D6 may last for many weeks after terbinafine is discontinued. Theoretically, because amiodarone inhibits both CYP2D6 and CYP3A4, it would be expected to markedly increase aripiprazole concentrations.

CLASS 3: ASSESS RISK & TAKE ACTION IF NECESSARY

- *Consider Alternative:*
  <u>Diphenhydramine</u>: Other antihistamines such as **desloratadine** (Clarinex), **fexofenadine** (Allegra), **loratadine** Claritin), and **cetirizine** (Zyrtec) are not known to inhibit CYP2D6.
  <u>Propoxyphene</u>: Consider using an alternative analgesic; propoxyphene has limited efficacy, and other analgesics appear less likely to affect CYP2D6.
- *Monitor:* Be alert for altered effect of aripiprazole if CYP2D6 inhibitors are started, stopped, or changed in dosage. Due to the long half-life of aripiprazole and its active metabolite, the onset and offset of these interactions may take one to two weeks.

OBJECT DRUGS	PRECIPITANT DRUGS
Aspirin	Ibuprofen

COMMENTS: Ibuprofen has been shown to interfere with the ability of aspirin to inhibit platelet aggregation, and some evidence suggests that this may also inhibit the cardioprotective effect of aspirin. The effect was seen when ibuprofen was given 2 hours before aspirin, and when ibuprofen was given in multiple doses. No effect on aspirin's antiplatelet effect was seen with a single ibuprofen dose 2 hours after the aspirin. Current evidence suggests that the antiplatelet effect of aspirin is not affected by diclofenac, and preliminary data suggest that the effect of other NSAIDs on aspirin is limited. Celecoxib (and probably other COX-2 inhibitors) and acetaminophen do not affect platelet function or the antiplatelet effect of aspirin.

CLASS 3: ASSESS RISK & TAKE ACTION IF NECESSARY
- *Consider Alternative*: Acetaminophen could be used as an analgesic in place of a NSAID. Consider using **diclofenac** (Voltaren) or a COX-2 inhibitor as an alternative anti-inflammatory agent. Higher analgesic doses of aspirin could be used without loss of antiplatelet effect. Until further data are available, one must consider the possibility that other NSAIDs could inhibit the antiplatelet effect of aspirin.
- *Circumvent/Minimize*: If the ibuprofen is only taken once daily, giving it 2 hours after the aspirin appears to minimize the interaction.

OBJECT DRUGS	PRECIPITANT DRUGS	
Azole Antifungals:	**Enzyme Inducers:**	
Itraconazole	**Barbiturates**	**Primidone** (Mysoline)
(Sporanox)	**Carbamazepine** (Tegretol)	**Rifabutin** (Mycobutin)
Ketoconazole (Nizoral)	**Efavirenz** (Sustiva)	**Rifampin** (Rifadin)
Posaconazole (Noxafil)	**Nevirapine** (Viramune)	**Rifapentine** (Priftin)
Voriconazole (Vfend)	**Oxcarbazepine** (Trileptal)	**St. John's Wort**
	Phenytoin (Dilantin)	

COMMENTS: Rifampin, carbamazepine, phenytoin (and probably other enzyme inducers) markedly reduce serum concentrations of these antifungals. Due to the large magnitude of the interaction it may be difficult to achieve therapeutic concentrations of these antifungal agents. The azole antifungals may also affect some of the enzyme inducers. For example, the azole antifungals may markedly increase carbamazepine or rifabutin concentrations, and voriconazole can increase efavirenz concentrations.

CLASS 3: ASSESS RISK & TAKE ACTION IF NECESSARY
- *Consider Alternative*:
  Antifungal Agent: **Fluconazole** (Diflucan) appears less likely to interact than other azole antifungals (because of its extensive renal elimination, it is less affected by enzyme inducers), but some reports suggest that enzyme inducers may also reduce fluconazole efficacy. In one study, rifampin markedly increased the clearance of **terbinafine** (Lamisil), so it may also interact.
- *Monitor*: Be alert for loss of antifungal efficacy, and consider increasing the dose of the azole antifungal. Keep in mind that enzyme induction is usually gradual and may take days to weeks for onset and offset, depending on the specific inducer.

OBJECT DRUGS	PRECIPITANT DRUGS	
Azole Antifungals:	**Gastric Antisecretory**	
Itraconazole (Sporanox)	**Agents:**	**Nizatidine** (Axid)
Ketoconazole (Nizoral)	**Cimetidine** (Tagamet)	**Omeprazole** (Prilosec)
	Deslansoprazole	**Pantoprazole** (Protonix)
	(Kapidex)	**Rabeprazole** (Aciphex)
	Esomeprazole (Nexium)	**Ranitidine** (Zantac)
	Famotidine (Pepcid)	
	Lansoprazole (Prevacid)	

COMMENTS: Itraconazole and ketoconazole require gastric acidity to be absorbed. Any agent that increases gastric pH can impair their bioavailability.

CLASS 3: ASSESS RISK & TAKE ACTION IF NECESSARY
- *Consider Alternative:* Consider **fluconazole** (Diflucan), **voriconazole** (Vfend), or **terbinafine** (Lamisil) if suitable for the infection.
- *Circumvent/Minimize:* The bioavailability of **itraconazole solution** is not affected by changes in gastric pH. If an antisecretory agent is necessary, consider using a larger dose of itraconazole or ketoconazole, with monitoring of antifungal serum concentrations if possible. The administration of the antifungal with **Coca-Cola** or **Pepsi** will acidify the stomach and improve the absorption of the antifungal; however a reduction in bioavailability will still occur.
- *Monitor:* Monitor for reduced antifungal effect if itraconazole or ketoconazole is used with a gastric alkalinizer or sucralfate.

OBJECT DRUGS	PRECIPITANT DRUGS
Azole Antifungals:	**Gastric Alkalinizers:**
Itraconazole (Sporanox)	**Antacids**
Ketoconazole (Nizoral)	**Didanosine** (Videx)
	Sucralfate (Carafate)

COMMENTS: Itraconazole and ketoconazole require gastric acidity to be absorbed. Any agent that increases gastric pH can impair their bioavailability. Sucralfate, although not strictly a gastric alkalinizer, has also been noted to reduce the absorption of itraconazole and ketoconazole.

CLASS 3: ASSESS RISK & TAKE ACTION IF NECESSARY
- *Consider Alternative:* Consider **fluconazole** (Diflucan), **voriconazole** (Vfend) or **terbinafine** (Lamisil) if suitable for the infection.
- *Circumvent/Minimize:* The bioavailability of **itraconazole solution** is not affected by changes in gastric pH. The interaction does not occur with enteric coated bead formulation of didanosine (Videx EC). Administer itraconazole or ketoconazole 2 or more hours prior to antacid, sucralfate, or didanosine. Wait six hours after gastric alkalinizer administration to give itraconazole or ketoconazole.
- *Monitor:* Monitor for reduced antifungal effect if itraconazole or ketoconazole is used with a gastric alkalinizer or sucralfate.

OBJECT DRUGS	PRECIPITANT DRUGS
Beta-blockers (Nonselective):	**Epinephrine** (Systemic doses)
Carteolol (Ocupress)	
Carvedilol (Coreg)	
Levobunolol (Betagan)	
Nadolol (Corgard)	
Penbutolol (Levatol)	
Pindolol (Visken)	
Propranolol (Inderal)	
Sotalol (Betapace)	
Timolol (Blocadren)	

COMMENTS: Non-cardioselective beta-blockers markedly increase the pressor response to epinephrine; this effect is not likely with epinephrine doses used for non-systemic effects (e.g., with local anesthetics) unless very large amounts are used. Patients prone to anaphylaxis should avoid all beta-blockers if possible (due to poor response to epinephrine should anaphylaxis occur). Ophthalmic use of beta-blockers can result in systemic beta-blockade in some patients.

CLASS 2: USE ONLY IF BENEFIT FELT TO OUTWEIGH RISK
- *Use Alternative*: Cardioselective beta-blockers are unlikely to result in hypertensive reactions in patients who receive systemic doses of epinephrine; thus, they are preferable to non-cardioselective beta-blockers if beta-blockers must be used. Cardioselective beta-blockers include **acebutolol** (Sectral), **atenolol** (Tenormin), **betaxolol** (Kerlone), **bisoprolol** (Zebeta), **esmolol** (Brevibloc), **metoprolol** (Lopressor), and **nebivolol** (Bystolic). Most cardioselective beta-blockers can become nonselective when used in large doses. Also, cardioselective agents that are metabolized by CYP2D6 such as metoprolol and nebivolol can become nonselective in people with reduced CYP2D6 activity, genetically or due to CYP2D6 inhibitors.

OBJECT DRUGS	PRECIPITANT DRUGS
Beta-blockers (CYP2D6 Substrates):	**Antidepressants:**
Carvedilol (Coreg)	**Bupropion** (Wellbutrin)
Metoprolol (Lopressor)	**Duloxetine** (Cymbalta)
Nebivolol (Bystolic)	**Fluoxetine** (Prozac)
Propranolol (Inderal)	**Paroxetine** (Paxil)
Timolol (Blocadren)	

COMMENTS: Antidepressants that are inhibitors of CYP2D6 can increase the concentration of beta-blockers, potentially resulting in bradycardia, hypotension or heart failure. Rapid metabolizers of CYP2D6 (over 90% of the population) will be at the greatest risk.

CLASS 3: ASSESS RISK & TAKE ACTION IF NECESSARY
- *Consider Alternative*:
  Antidepressant: **Sertraline** (Zoloft), **citalopram** (Celexa), **desvenlafaxine** (Pristiq), and **escitalopram** (Lexapro) are weak inhibitors of CYP2D6, while

venlafaxine (Effexor) and **fluvoxamine** (Luvox) have little or no effect on CYP2D6.

Beta-blocker: Select a beta-blocker that is not a CYP2D6 substrate such as **atenolol** (Tenormin) or **nadolol** (Corgard).

- *Monitor*: Monitor for altered beta-blocker effect if inhibitor is initiated, discontinued, or changed in dosage.

OBJECT DRUGS	PRECIPITANT DRUGS
Beta-blockers	**Enzyme Inhibitors:**
(CYP2D6 Substrates):	**Amiodarone** (Cordarone)
Carvedilol (Coreg)	**Cimetidine** (Tagamet)
Metoprolol (Lopressor)	**Cinacalcet** (Sensipar)
Nebivolol (Bystolic)	**Diphenhydramine** (Benadryl)
Propranolol (Inderal)	**Haloperidol** (Haldol)
Timolol (Blocadren)	**Propafenone** (Rythmol)
	Propoxyphene (Darvon)
	Quinidine (Quinidex)
	Ritonavir (Norvir)
	Terbinafine (Lamisil)
	Thioridazine (Mellaril)

COMMENTS: Inhibitors of CYP2D6 can increase the concentration of beta-blockers, potentially resulting in bradycardia, hypotension or heart failure. Rapid metabolizers of CYP2D6 (over 90% of the population) will be at the greatest risk. Note that because terbinafine has an extraordinarily long terminal half-life, the inhibitory effect of terbinafine on CYP2D6 may last for many weeks after terbinafine is discontinued.

CLASS 3: ASSESS RISK & TAKE ACTION IF NECESSARY

- *Consider Alternative*:
  Cimetidine: Other acid suppressors are unlikely to interact. Consider using **famotidine** (Pepcid), **nizatidine** (Axid), **ranitidine** (Zantac), **deslansoprazole** (Kapidex), **esomeprazole** (Nexium), **omeprazole** (Prilosec), **lansoprazole** (Prevacid), **rabeprazole** (Aciphex), or **pantoprazole** (Protonix).
  Beta-blocker: Select a beta-blocker that is not a CYP2D6 substrate such as **atenolol** (Tenormin) or **nadolol** (Corgard).
- *Monitor*: Monitor for altered beta-blocker effect if inhibitor is initiated, discontinued, or changed in dosage.

OBJECT DRUGS	PRECIPITANT DRUGS
Calcium Channel Blockers:	**Enzyme Inducers:**
Amlodipine (Norvasc)	**Barbiturates**
Bepridil (Vascor)	**Carbamazepine** (Tegretol)
Diltiazem (Cardizem)	**Efavirenz** (Sustiva)
Felodipine (Plendil)	**Nafcillin** (Unipen)
Isradipine (DynaCirc)	**Nevirapine** (Viramune)
Nicardipine (Cardene)	**Oxcarbazepine** (Trileptal)
Nifedipine (Procardia)	**Phenytoin** (Dilantin)
Nimodipine (Nimotop)	**Primidone** (Mysoline)
Nisoldipine (Sular)	**Rifabutin** (Mycobutin)
Nitrendipine (Baypress)	**Rifampin** (Rifadin)
Verapamil (Isoptin)	**Rifapentine** (Priftin)
	St. John's Wort

COMMENTS: Rifampin markedly reduces the plasma concentrations of verapamil, diltiazem, nifedipine, and nisoldipine; the effect probably occurs with most other combinations of calcium channel blockers (CCBs) and enzyme inducers. The effect is greater with oral than with parenteral administration of the CCB.

CLASS 3: ASSESS RISK & TAKE ACTION IF NECESSARY

- *Consider Alternative:* It may be difficult to achieve therapeutic serum concentrations of oral CCBs in the presence of enzyme inducers. Thus, if at all possible, use an alternative to either the CCB or the enzyme inducer. Avoid barbiturates if a non-barbiturate alternative is suitable (e.g., benzodiazepine). Theoretically, amlodipine would be less affected than other CCBs, since it undergoes less first-pass metabolism.
- *Monitor:* Monitor for altered CCB effect if inducer is initiated, discontinued, or changed in dosage. Keep in mind that enzyme induction is usually gradual and may take days to weeks for onset and offset, depending on the specific inducer.

OBJECT DRUGS		PRECIPITANT DRUGS
Calcium Channel Blockers:		**Antidepressants:**
	Nicardipine (Cardene)	**Fluvoxamine** (Luvox)
Amlodipine (Norvasc)	**Nifedipine** (Procardia)	**Nefazodone**
Bepridil (Vascor)	**Nimodipine** (Nimotop)	
Diltiazem (Cardizem)	**Nisoldipine** (Sular)	
Felodipine (Plendil)	**Nitrendipine** (Baypress)	
Isradipine (DynaCirc)	**Verapamil** (Isoptin)	

COMMENTS: CYP3A4 inhibitors may substantially increase calcium channel blocker (CCB) serum concentrations. Not all combinations of CCBs and CYP3A4 inhibitors have been studied; assume they interact until proven otherwise. Note, however, that the magnitude of interaction can vary considerably depending on the CCB involved. For example, felodipine undergoes extensive first pass metabolism by CYP3A4 and is markedly affected by CYP3A4 inhibition, while amlodipine undergoes considerably less first pass metabolism by CYP3A4 and is much less affected by CYP3A4 inhibition. Fluvoxamine appears to be a modest CYP3A4 inhibitor but may produce increased CCB concentrations.

CLASS 3: ASSESS RISK & TAKE ACTION IF NECESSARY
- *Consider Alternative*: **Sertraline** (Zoloft), **citalopram** (Celexa), **escitalopram** (Lexapro), **desvenlafaxine** (Pristiq), **venlafaxine** (Effexor), and **paroxetine** (Paxil) appear less likely to inhibit CYP3A4 than fluvoxamine. Little is known about the effect of other antidepressants on CCBs.
- *Monitor*: If alternatives are not appropriate, consider reducing CCB dose and monitor for altered CCB response if inhibitor is initiated, discontinued, or changed in dosage.

OBJECT DRUGS	PRECIPITANT DRUGS
Calcium Channel Blockers:	**Antimicrobials:**
Amlodipine (Norvasc)	**Clarithromycin** (Biaxin)
Bepridil (Vascor)	**Erythromycin** (E-Mycin)
Diltiazem (Cardizem)	**Fluconazole** (Diflucan)
Felodipine (Plendil)	**Itraconazole** (Sporanox)
Isradipine (DynaCirc)	**Ketoconazole** (Nizoral)
Nicardipine (Cardene)	**Posaconazole** (Noxafil)
Nifedipine (Procardia)	**Quinupristin** (Synercid)
Nimodipine (Nimotop)	**Telithromycin** (Ketek)
Nisoldipine (Sular)	**Troleandomycin** (TAO)
Nitrendipine (Baypress)	**Voriconazole** (Vfend)
Verapamil (Isoptin)	

COMMENTS: Calcium channel blockers (CCBs) are metabolized by CYP3A4, so CYP3A4 inhibitors may substantially increase their serum concentrations. Not all combinations of CCBs and CYP3A4 inhibitors have been studied; assume they interact until proven otherwise. Note, however, that the magnitude of interaction can vary considerably depending on the CCB involved. For example, felodipine undergoes extensive first pass metabolism by CYP3A4 and is markedly affected by CYP3A4 inhibition, while amlodipine undergoes considerably less first pass metabolism by CYP3A4 and is much less affected by CYP3A4 inhibition. Short-term use of an azole antifungal (1-2 days) is unlikely to result in a clinically important interaction.

CLASS 3: ASSESS RISK & TAKE ACTION IF NECESSARY
- *Consider Alternative*:
  Azole Antifungals: Fluconazole appears to be a less potent inhibitor of CYP3A4; but in larger doses it also inhibits CYP3A4. **Terbinafine** (Lamisil) does not appear to affect CYP3A4.
  Macrolide Antibiotics: Unlike erythromycin, clarithromycin and troleandomycin, **azithromycin** (Zithromax) and **dirithromycin*** do not appear to inhibit CYP3A4. (*not available in US)
  Telithromycin: The use of **azithromycin** (Zithromax) or a quinolone antibiotic should be considered.

- *Monitor*: If alternatives are not appropriate, consider reducing CCB dose and monitor for altered CCB response if inhibitor is initiated, discontinued, or changed in dosage.

OBJECT DRUGS	PRECIPITANT DRUGS	
Calcium Channel Blockers:	**Enzyme Inhibitors:**	
Amlodipine (Norvasc)	**Amiodarone** (Cordarone)	**Grapefruit**
Bepridil (Vascor)	**Amprenavir** (Agenerase)	**Indinavir** (Crixivan)
Diltiazem (Cardizem)	**Aprepitant** (Emend)	**Nelfinavir** (Viracept)
Felodipine (Plendil)	**Atazanavir** (Reyataz)	**Ritonavir** (Norvir)
Isradipine (DynaCirc)	**Conivaptan** (Vaprisol)	**Saquinavir** (Invirase)
Nicardipine (Cardene)	**Cyclosporine** (Neoral)	**Verapamil** (Isoptin)
Nifedipine (Procardia)	**Darunavir** (Prezista)	
Nimodipine (Nimotop)	**Delavirdine** (Rescriptor)	
Nisoldipine (Sular)	**Diltiazem** (Cardizem)	
Nitrendipine (Baypress)		
Verapamil (Isoptin)		

COMMENTS: Calcium channel blockers (CCBs) are metabolized by CYP3A4, so CYP3A4 inhibitors may substantially increase their serum concentrations. Not all combinations of CCBs and CYP3A4 inhibitors have been studied; assume they interact until proven otherwise. Note, however, that the magnitude of interaction can vary considerably depending on the CCB involved. For example, felodipine undergoes extensive first pass metabolism by CYP3A4 and is markedly affected by CYP3A4 inhibition, while amlodipine undergoes considerably less first pass metabolism by CYP3A4 and is much less affected by CYP3A4 inhibition. For example, grapefruit juice substantially increases felodipine concentrations, but has minimal effects on amlodipine.

CLASS 3: ASSESS RISK & TAKE ACTION IF NECESSARY
- *Monitor*: If alternatives are not appropriate, consider reducing CCB dose and monitor for altered CCB response if inhibitor is initiated, discontinued, or changed in dosage.

OBJECT DRUGS	PRECIPITANT DRUGS
Carbamazepine (Tegretol)	**Antidepressants:**
	Fluoxetine (Prozac)
	Fluvoxamine (Luvox)
	Nefazodone

COMMENTS: Inhibition of CYP3A4 by fluvoxamine may result in carbamazepine toxicity. As with most CYP3A4 inhibitors, carbamazepine toxicity usually occurs within 2-3 days of starting the inhibitor. The effect of fluoxetine on carbamazepine is less consistent and may be delayed by 1-2 weeks or longer; it may involve enzymes in addition to CYP3A4, perhaps CYP2C19. Nefazodone is a potent CYP3A4 inhibitor and would be expected to produce marked increases in carbamazepine concentrations in most patients.

- **Consider Alternative**: **Sertraline** (Zoloft), **citalopram** (Celexa), **escitalopram** (Lexapro), **venlafaxine** (Effexor), and **paroxetine** (Paxil) appear less likely to inhibit CYP3A4 than fluvoxamine. Little is known about the effects of other antidepressants on carbamazepine.
- **Monitor**: If alternatives are not appropriate, consider reducing dose of carbamazepine. Monitor for altered carbamazepine effect if enzyme inhibitors are initiated, discontinued, or changed in dosage. Symptoms of carbamazepine toxicity include nausea, vomiting, dizziness, drowsiness, headache, diplopia, and confusion.

OBJECT DRUGS	PRECIPITANT DRUGS	
Carbamazepine (Tegretol)	**Antimicrobials:**	
	Clarithromycin (Biaxin)	**Posaconazole** (Noxafil)
	Erythromycin (E-Mycin)	**Quinupristin** (Synercid)
	Fluconazole (Diflucan)	**Telithromycin** (Ketek)
	Itraconazole (Sporanox)	**Troleandomycin** (TAO)
	Ketoconazole (Nizoral)	**Voriconazole** (Vfend)

COMMENTS: Inhibition of CYP3A4 by these antimicrobials may result in carbamazepine toxicity, usually within 2-3 days of starting the inhibitor. Adverse outcomes from these interactions are fairly predictable, and most patients who start a CYP3A4 inhibitor while on carbamazepine will develop clinical evidence of carbamazepine toxicity. **Metronidazole** (Flagyl) has also been reported to cause carbamazepine toxicity in isolated cases, but more study is needed.

CLASS 3: ASSESS RISK & TAKE ACTION IF NECESSARY
- **Consider Alternative**:
  Azole Antifungals: Fluconazole appears to be a less potent inhibitor of CYP3A4; but in larger doses it also inhibits CYP3A4. **Terbinafine** (Lamisil) does not appear to affect CYP3A4.
  Macrolide Antibiotics: Unlike erythromycin, clarithromycin and troleandomycin, **azithromycin** (Zithromax) and **dirithromycin*** do not appear to inhibit CYP3A4. (*not available in US)
  Telithromycin: The use of **azithromycin** (Zithromax) or a quinolone antibiotic should be considered.
- **Monitor**: If alternatives are not appropriate, consider reducing dose of carbamazepine. Monitor for altered carbamazepine effect if enzyme inhibitors are initiated, discontinued, or changed in dosage. Symptoms of carbamazepine toxicity include nausea, vomiting, dizziness, drowsiness, headache, diplopia, and confusion.

OBJECT DRUGS	PRECIPITANT DRUGS
Carbamazepine (Tegretol)	**Calcium Channel Blockers:**
	Diltiazem (Cardizem)
	Verapamil (Isoptin)

COMMENTS: Inhibition of CYP3A4 by these calcium channel blockers may result in carbamazepine toxicity, usually within 2-3 days of starting the inhibitor.

Adverse outcomes from these interactions are fairly predictable, and most patients who start a CYP3A4 inhibitor while on carbamazepine will develop clinical evidence of carbamazepine toxicity. Keep in mind also that enzyme inducers such as carbamazepine can markedly reduce plasma concentrations of most calcium channel blockers.

CLASS 3: ASSESS RISK & TAKE ACTION IF NECESSARY

- *Consider Alternative*: Diltiazem, verapamil, and possibly nicardipine are the only calcium channel blockers (CCBs) known to inhibit CYP3A4; other CCBs are probably less likely to cause carbamazepine toxicity.
- *Monitor*: If alternatives are not appropriate, consider reducing dose of carbamazepine. Monitor for altered carbamazepine effect if enzyme inhibitors are initiated, discontinued, or changed in dosage. Symptoms of carbamazepine toxicity include nausea, vomiting, dizziness, drowsiness, headache, diplopia, and confusion.

OBJECT DRUGS	PRECIPITANT DRUGS	
Carbamazepine (Tegretol)	**Enzyme Inhibitors:**	
	Amiodarone (Cordarone)	**Grapefruit**
	Amprenavir (Agenerase)	**Indinavir** (Crixivan)
	Aprepitant (Emend)	**Isoniazid** (INH)
	Atazanavir (Reyataz)	**Nelfinavir** (Viracept)
	Cimetidine (Tagamet)	**Propoxyphene** (Darvon)
	Conivaptan (Vaprisol)	**Ritonavir** (Norvir)
	Cyclosporine (Neoral)	**Saquinavir** (Invirase)
	Danazol (Danocrine)	
	Darunavir (Prezista)	
	Delavirdine (Rescriptor)	

COMMENTS: Inhibition of CYP3A4 may result in carbamazepine toxicity, usually within 2-3 days of starting the inhibitor. Adverse outcomes from these interactions are fairly predictable, and most patients who start a CYP3A4 inhibitor while on carbamazepine will develop clinical evidence of carbamazepine toxicity. The effect of danazol may be delayed by 1-2 weeks. Not all known CYP3A4 inhibitors have been studied with carbamazepine, but assume they interact until proven otherwise.

CLASS 3: ASSESS RISK & TAKE ACTION IF NECESSARY

- *Consider Alternative*:
  Cimetidine: **Famotidine** (Pepcid), **nizatidine** (Axid), and **ranitidine** (Zantac) have minimal effects on drug metabolism.
  Grapefruit: Orange juice does not appear to inhibit CYP3A4.
- *Monitor*: If alternatives are not appropriate, consider reducing dose of carbamazepine. Monitor for altered carbamazepine effect if enzyme inhibitors are initiated, discontinued, or changed in dosage. Symptoms of carbamazepine toxicity include nausea, vomiting, dizziness, drowsiness, headache, diplopia, and confusion.

OBJECT DRUGS	PRECIPITANT DRUGS	
Central Alpha-adrenergic Agonists:	**Antidepressants, Tricyclic:**	
Clonidine (Catapres)	**Amitriptyline** (Elavil)	**Imipramine** (Tofranil)
Guanabenz (Wytensin)	**Amoxapine** (Asendin)	**Mirtazapine** (Remeron)
Guanfacine (Tenex)	**Clomipramine** (Anafranil)	**Nortriptyline** (Aventyl)
	Desipramine (Norpramin)	**Protriptyline** (Vivactil)
	Doxepin (Sinequan)	**Trimipramine** (Surmontil)

COMMENTS: Tricyclic antidepressants (TCAs) can markedly reduce the antihypertensive effects of clonidine, guanfacine, and probably guanabenz. The effect is usually gradual but rapid increases in blood pressure have occurred. Also, stopping clonidine-like drugs abruptly in the presence of TCAs may result in an acute hypertensive reaction. Several case reports suggest that **chlorpromazine** may also inhibit the antihypertensive response to guanethidine, but more study is needed.

CLASS 2: USE ONLY IF BENEFIT FELT TO OUTWEIGH RISK
- *Use Alternative*:
  Antidepressant: Limited evidence suggests that **trazodone** (Desyrel) may inhibit the effect of clonidine, but little is known regarding the effect of other antidepressants on clonidine-like drugs. Use alternative antidepressants only with careful blood pressure monitoring.
  Antihypertensives: Beta-adrenergic blockers, diuretics, ACEIs, ARBs, and calcium channel blockers appear to be minimally affected by TCAs. Be alert to the potential for **diltiazem** (Cardizem) and **verapamil** (Calan) to inhibit the metabolism of some TCAs. The efficacy of **guanethidine** (Ismelin) and **guanadrel** (Hylorel) is also inhibited by TCAs.
- *Circumvent/Minimize:* In patients receiving central alpha agonists and TCAs, clonidine-like drugs should be tapered instead of stopped abruptly to reduce the likelihood of a hypertensive reaction.
- *Monitor:* In patients on central alpha-receptor agonists, monitor blood pressure carefully if TCAs are initiated, discontinued, or changed in dosage.

OBJECT DRUGS	PRECIPITANT DRUGS	
Cephalosporin Antibiotics:	**Gastric Alkalinizers:**	
Cefditoren (Spectracef)	**Antacids**	**Nizatidine** (Axid)
Cefpodoxime (Vantin)	**Cimetidine** (Tagamet)	**Omeprazole** (Prilosec)
Cefuroxime (Ceftin)	**Deslansoprazole** (Kapidex)	**Pantoprazole** (Protonix)
	Esomeprazole (Nexium)	**Rabeprazole** (Aciphex)
	Famotidine (Pepcid)	**Ranitidine** (Zantac)
	Lansoprazole (Prevacid)	

COMMENTS: Increasing gastric pH inhibits the absorption of cefditoren, cefpodoxime, and cefuroxime. A loss of efficacy could result.

CLASS 3: ASSESS RISK & TAKE ACTION IF NECESSARY

Circumvent/Minimize: Administration of the cephalosporin 2 hours before the antacid would minimize the interaction. It may be difficult to separate the doses of an H_2-receptor antagonist or proton pump inhibitor to ensure that no interaction occurs.

- *Consider Alternative:* H_2-receptor antagonists do not affect **cefixime** (Suprax) absorption; theoretically it would also be unaffected by proton pump inhibitors. Other cephalosporins are not known to manifest pH-dependent absorption.
- *Monitor:* Watch for reduced antibiotic efficacy when these cephalosporins are coadministered with gastric alkalinizers.

OBJECT DRUGS	PRECIPITANT DRUGS
Clozapine (Clozaril) **Olanzapine** (Zyprexa)	**Fluvoxamine** (Luvox)

COMMENTS: Agents that inhibit CYP1A2 and possibly CYP2C19 increase clozapine and olanzapine plasma levels. Fluvoxamine has a marked effect, and can increase serum clozapine concentrations up to 5-10 fold. Fluvoxamine has been used to increase clozapine efficacy in patients with resistant schizophrenia, but careful monitoring is necessary to avoid clozapine toxicity. Some other SSRIs may produce modest increases in clozapine plasma concentrations, including **fluoxetine**, **paroxetine** and **sertraline**.

CLASS 2: USE ONLY IF BENEFIT FELT TO OUTWEIGH RISK

- *Use Alternative:* Fluoxetine (Prozac), **paroxetine** (Paxil), and **sertraline** (Zoloft) appear to interact less than fluvoxamine. Theoretically, **venlafaxine** (Effexor) would be even less likely to interact, but information is lacking.
- *Monitor:* Monitor for altered clozapine or olanzapine response if a CYP1A2 inhibitor such as fluvoxamine is initiated, discontinued, or dose is changed.

OBJECT DRUGS	PRECIPITANT DRUGS	
Clozapine (Clozaril) **Olanzapine** (Zyprexa)	**Enzyme Inhibitors:**	
	Atazanavir (Reyataz)	**Enoxacin** (Penetrex)
	Cimetidine (Tagamet)	**Mexiletine** (Mexitil)
	Ciprofloxacin (Cipro)	**Tacrine** (Cognex)
	Contraceptives, Oral	**Zileuton** (Zyflo)

COMMENTS: Agents that inhibit CYP1A2 and possibly CYP2C19 increase clozapine and olanzapine plasma levels. **Enoxacin** is a potent inhibitor of CYP1A2 and would be expected to markedly increase clozapine and olanzapine plasma concentrations; it should be considered a **Class 2** interaction. Oral contraceptives are generally modest inhibitors of CYP1A2, and the degree of inhibition is likely to be highly variable depending on the dose of the contraceptive and specific patient characteristics.

CLASS 3: ASSESS RISK & TAKE ACTION IF NECESSARY

- *Consider Alternative:*
  Cimetidine: **Famotidine** (Pepcid), **nizatidine** (Axid), and **ranitidine** (Zantac) have minimal effects on drug metabolism.

Ciprofloxacin or Enoxacin: **Gemifloxacin** (Factive), **levofloxacin** (Levaquin), **lomefloxacin** (Maxaquin), **moxifloxacin** (Avelox), and **ofloxacin** (Floxin), appear to have little effect on CYP1A2.

- *Monitor*: Monitor for altered clozapine or olanzapine response if a CYP1A2 inhibitor is initiated, discontinued, or dose is changed.

OBJECT DRUGS	PRECIPITANT DRUGS
Codeine Derivatives:	**Antidepressants:**
Codeine	**Bupropion** (Wellbutrin)
Dihydrocodeine (Synalgos-DC)	**Duloxetine** (Cymbalta)
Hydrocodone (Vicodin, Lortab)	**Fluoxetine** (Prozac)
	Paroxetine (Paxil)

COMMENTS: Antidepressants that inhibit CYP2D6 prevent the conversion of codeine to its active metabolite, morphine; inhibition of analgesic effect may result. Preliminary evidence suggests that the analgesic effect of hydrocodone and dihydrocodeine is also reduced in the absence of CYP2D6 activity. The analgesic effect of **tramadol** (Ultram) appears to be only partially dependent on CYP2D6, and thus it may have some analgesic activity in the presence of CYP2D6 inhibitors.

CLASS 3: ASSESS RISK & TAKE ACTION IF NECESSARY

- *Consider Alternative*:
  Analgesic: Consider using an analgesic that does not require conversion to an active metabolite, e.g., **morphine**, **methadone** (Dolophine), **fentanyl** (Duragesic), **hydromorphone** (Dilaudid), **butorphanol** (Stadol), or **oxymorphone** (Numorphan). Preliminary evidence suggests that **oxycodone** (Percodan, Percocet) may not require CYP2D6 for activity.
  Antidepressant: **Citalopram** (Celexa), **escitalopram** (Lexapro), and **sertraline** (Zoloft) are weak inhibitors of CYP2D6, **desvenlafaxine** (Pristiq), **venlafaxine** (Effexor) and **fluvoxamine** (Luvox) have little or no effect on CYP2D6
- *Monitor*: Monitor for loss of analgesic efficacy.

OBJECT DRUGS	PRECIPITANT DRUGS	
Codeine Derivatives:	**Enzyme Inhibitors:**	
Codeine	**Amiodarone** (Cordarone)	**Propafenone** (Rythmol)
Dihydrocodeine	**Cimetidine** (Tagamet)	**Propoxyphene** (Darvon)
(Synalgos-DC)	**Cinacalcet** (Sensipar)	**Quinidine** (Quinidex)
Hydrocodone (Vicodin,	**Diphenhydramine**	**Ritonavir** (Norvir)
Lortab)	(Benadryl)	**Terbinafine** (Lamisil)
	Haloperidol (Haldol)	**Thioridazine** (Mellaril)

COMMENTS: Inhibitors of CYP2D6 prevent the conversion of codeine to its active metabolite, morphine; inhibition of analgesic effect may result. Preliminary evidence suggests that the analgesic effect of hydrocodone and dihydrocodeine is also reduced in the absence of CYP2D6 activity. The analgesic effect of **tramadol** (Ultram) appears to be only partially dependent on CYP2D6, and thus it may have some analgesic activity in the presence of CYP2D6 inhibitors. Note that because terbinafine has an extraordinarily long terminal half-life, the inhibitory effect of terbinafine on CYP2D6 may last for many weeks after terbinafine is discontinued.

CLASS 3: ASSESS RISK & TAKE ACTION IF NECESSARY

- *Consider Alternative*:
  Analgesic: Consider using an analgesic that does not require conversion to an active metabolite, e.g., **morphine**, **methadone** (Dolophine), **fentanyl** (Duragesic), **hydromorphone** (Dilaudid), **butorphanol** (Stadol), or **oxymorphone** (Numorphan). Preliminary evidence suggests that **oxycodone** (Percodan, Percocet) may not require CYP2D6 for activity.
  Cimetidine: Other H_2-receptor antagonists such as **famotidine** (Pepcid), **nizatidine** (Axid), or **ranitidine** (Zantac) may be substituted for cimetidine.
- *Monitor*: Monitor for loss of analgesic efficacy.

OBJECT DRUGS	PRECIPITANT DRUGS	
Colchicine	**Antimicrobials:**	
	Clarithromycin (Biaxin)	**Posaconazole** (Noxafil)
	Erythromycin (E-Mycin)	**Quinupristin** (Synercid)
	Fluconazole (Diflucan)	**Telithromycin** (Ketek)
	Itraconazole (Sporanox)	**Troleandomycin** (TAO)
	Ketoconazole (Nizoral)	**Voriconazole** (Vfend)

COMMENTS: Colchicine is a substrate for P-glycoprotein (PGP) and concurrent use of PGP inhibitors has resulted in severe colchicine toxicity. Colchicine is also a substrate for CYP3A4 and inhibitors of this enzyme may also increase its plasma concentrations.

CLASS 2: USE ONLY IF BENEFIT FELT TO OUTWEIGH RISK

- *Use Alternative*: Given the possibility of fatal colchicine toxicity, few situations would warrant the use of a PGP or CYP3A4 inhibitor with colchicine. Select an alternative that is not known to inhibit PGP or CYP3A4, especially if the patient has renal impairment.
  Azole Antifungals: **Terbinafine** (Lamisil) does not appear to affect CYP3A4, and is not known to inhibit P-glycoprotein, but monitor for colchicine toxicity if it is used.
  Macrolide Antibiotics: Unlike erythromycin, clarithromycin and troleandomycin, **azithromycin** (Zithromax) does not appear to inhibit CYP3A4. But it may weakly inhibit P-glycoprotein, so monitor for colchicine toxicity if it is used.
- *Monitor*: If the combination must be used, monitor carefully for toxicity from colchicine including diarrhea, fever, abdominal pain, muscle pain or weakness, and paresthesias. Discontinue both drugs immediately if toxicity is suspected.

OBJECT DRUGS	PRECIPITANT DRUGS	
Colchicine	**P-glycoprotein and CYP3A4**	
	Inhibitors:	**Lapatinib** (Tykerb)
	Amiodarone (Cordarone)	**Nefazodone**
	Aprepitant (Emend)	**Nelfinavir** (Viracept)
	Atazanavir (Reyataz)	**Nicardipine** (Cardene)
	Conivaptan (Vaprisol)	**Propafenone** (Rythmol)
	Cyclosporine (Neoral)	**Quinidine** (Quinidex)
	Delavirdine (Rescriptor)	**Ritonavir** (Norvir)
	Diltiazem (Cardizem)	**Saquinavir** (Invirase)
	Dronedarone (Multaq)	**Tacrolimus** (Prograf)
	Grapefruit	**Tamoxifen** (Nolvadex)
	Indinavir (Crixivan)	**Verapamil** (Isoptin)

COMMENTS: Colchicine is a substrate for P-glycoprotein (PGP) and concurrent use of PGP inhibitors has resulted in severe colchicines toxicity. Colchicine is also a substrate for CYP3A4 and inhibitors of this enzyme may also raise its plasma concentrations. Grapefruit inhbits both CYP3A4 and PGP, and colchicine toxicity has been reported with intake of large amounts of grapefruit juice.

CLASS 2: USE ONLY IF BENEFIT FELT TO OUTWEIGH RISK
- *Use Alternative*: Given the possibility of fatal colchicine toxicity, few situations would warrant the use of a PGP or CYP3A4 inhibitor with colchicine. Select an alternative that is not known to inhibit PGP or CYP3A4, especially if the patient has renal impairment.
  Calcium Channel Blockers: Calcium channel blockers other than diltiazem, nicardipine, and verapamil appear less likely to inhibit CYP3A4, and may be less likely to inhibit P-glycoprotein. But monitor for colchicine toxicity if any calcium channel blocker is used concurrently.
  Grapefruit: Orange juice does not appear to inhibit CYP3A4.
- *Monitor*: If the combination must be used, monitor carefully for toxicity from colchicine including diarrhea, fever, abdominal pain, muscle pain or weakness, and paresthesias. Discontinue both drugs immediately if toxicity is suspected.

OBJECT DRUGS	PRECIPITANT DRUGS	
Contraceptives, Oral	**Enzyme Inducers:**	
	Barbiturates	**Oxcarbazepine** (Trileptal)
	Bexarotene (Targretin)	**Phenytoin** (Dilantin)
	Bosentan (Tracleer)	**Primidone** (Mysoline)
	Carbamazepine (Tegretol)	**Rifabutin** (Mycobutin)
	Efavirenz (Sustiva)	**Rifampin** (Rifadin)
	Felbamate (Felbatol)	**Rifapentine** (Priftin)
	Griseofulvin (Fulvicin)	**Ritonavir** (Norvir)
	Modafinil (Provigil)	**St. John's Wort**
	Nevirapine (Viramune)	**Topiramate** (Topamax)

COMMENTS: Enzyme inducers increase the risk of ovulation and unintended pregnancy in women receiving oral contraceptives. Felbamate may reduce levels of gestodene but not ethinyl estradiol. Bexarotene and bosentan are both known teratogens. At least one case of unintended pregnancy has been reported in a patient using an implantable hormonal contraceptive (Implanon) who took carbamazepine concurrently. The effect of modafinil appears modest, but could increase the risk of contraceptive failure in some people. Keep in mind that enzyme induction is usually gradual and may take days to weeks for onset and offset, depending on the specific inducer.

CLASS 2: USE ONLY IF BENEFIT FELT TO OUTWEIGH RISK

- *Use Alternative:* Use an alternative to the enzyme inducer if possible. If the enzyme inducer is necessary consider adding alternative contraception. <u>Anticonvulsants</u>: Agents that may be less likely to interact with oral contraceptives include **gabapentin** (Neurontin), **lamotrigine** (Lamictal), **pregabalin** (Lyrica), **tiagabine** (Gabitril), and **valproate** (Depakote).
- *Circumvent/Minimize:* If enzyme inducers are used with oral contraceptives, contraceptive dose may need to be increased. Nonetheless, increases in oral contraceptive dose do not guarantee contraceptive efficacy.
- *Monitor:* Menstrual irregularities (spotting, breakthrough bleeding) may be a sign of inadequate contraceptive hormone levels, but absence of menstrual problems does not guarantee adequate contraception.

OBJECT DRUGS	PRECIPITANT DRUGS
Contraceptives, Oral	<u>Antibiotics, Oral:</u>
	Amoxicillin (Amoxil)
	Ampicillin
	Tetracyclines
	Other Oral Antibiotics

COMMENTS: (See Contraceptives, Oral + Enzyme Inducers for rifabutin, rifapentine, and rifampin). Menstrual irregularities and (rarely) unintended pregnancies have occurred during or after oral antibiotic therapy in women on oral contraceptives. The antibiotics most often implicated are ampicillin (and related penicillins) and tetracyclines, but isolated cases have occurred with many antibiotics. Although a causal relationship has not been established, assume that the interaction occurs until proven otherwise. Theoretically antibiotics that inhibit CYP3A4 (e.g., erythromycin or clarithromycin) would inhibit estrogen and progestin metabolism, thus decreasing the likelihood of reduced contraceptive efficacy.

CLASS 3: ASSESS RISK & TAKE ACTION IF NECESSARY

- *Circumvent/Minimize:* Patients receiving oral contraceptives should be warned about the possibility of reduced efficacy if oral antibiotics are taken. It would be prudent to add other contraception during antibiotic therapy and for at least one cycle after the antibiotic is discontinued.
- *Monitor:* Menstrual irregularities (spotting, breakthrough bleeding) may be a sign of inadequate contraceptive hormone levels, but absence of menstrual problems does not guarantee adequate contraception.

OBJECT DRUGS	PRECIPITANT DRUGS
Corticosteroids:	**Antimicrobials:**
Budesonide (Entocort, Pulmicort)	**Clarithromycin** (Biaxin)
Dexamethasone (Decadron)	**Erythromycin** (E-Mycin)
Fluticasone (Flovent)	**Fluconazole** (Diflucan)
Methylprednisolone (Medrol)	**Itraconazole** (Sporanox)
	Ketoconazole (Nizoral)
	Posaconazole (Noxafil)
	Telithromycin (Ketek)
	Troleandomycin (TAO)
	Voriconazole (Vfend)

COMMENTS: Inhibition of CYP3A4 by these antimicrobials may result insubstantial increases in the plasma concentrations of these corticosteroids. This can lead to Cushing's syndrome and adrenal suppression. Although inhaled budesonide or fluticasone are not intended to act systemically, numerous cases have been reported of Cushing's syndrome and adrenal insufficiency due to concurrent use of potent CYP3A4 inhibitors such as itraconazole and ritonavir.

CLASS 3: ASSESS RISK & TAKE ACTION IF NECESSARY

- *Consider Alternative:*
  Corticosteroids: Clinical evidence suggests that prednisone and prednisolone are less affected by CYP3A4 inhibitors, but one should still be alert for evidence of corticosteroid toxicity. Theoretically, beclomethasone is unlikely to be affected by CYP3A4 inhibitors.
  Azole Antifungals: Itraconazole and ketoconazole are potent inhibitors of CYP3A4; fluconazole appears weaker, but in larger doses it also inhibits CYP3A4. **Terbinafine** (Lamisil) does not appear to affect CYP3A4, and would not be expected to interact with corticosteroids.
  Macrolide Antibiotics: Unlike erythromycin, clarithromycin and troleandomycin, **azithromycin** (Zithromax) and **dirithromycin*** do not appear to inhibit CYP3A4. (*not available in US)
- *Monitor:* If CYP3A4 inhibitors are used with dexamethasone or methylprednisolone, monitor for evidence of corticosteroid toxicity such as hypertension, edema, diabetes, myopathy, ocular toxicity, and Cushing's syndrome (moon face, central obesity, bruising, hirsutism, acne).

OBJECT DRUGS	PRECIPITANT DRUGS
Corticosteroids:	**Antidepressants:**
Budesonide (Entocort, Pulmicort)	**Fluvoxamine** (Luvox)
Dexamethasone (Decadron)	**Nefazodone**
Fluticasone (Flovent)	
Methylprednisolone (Medrol)	

COMMENTS: Inhibition of CYP3A4 by these antidepressants may result insubstantial increases in the plasma concentrations of these corticosteroids. This can lead to Cushing's syndrome and adrenal suppression. Although inhaled budesonide or fluticasone are not intended to act systemically, numerous cases have been reported of Cushing's syndrome and adrenal insufficiency due to concurrent use of potent CYP3A4.

CLASS 3: ASSESS RISK & TAKE ACTION IF NECESSARY

- *Consider Alternative*:

  Corticosteroids: Clinical evidence suggests that prednisone and prednisolone are less affected by CYP3A4 inhibitors, but one should still be alert for evidence of corticosteroid toxicity. Theoretically, beclomethasone is unlikely to be affected by CYP3A4 inhibitors.

  Antidepressants: **Sertraline** (Zoloft), **citalopram** (Celexa), **escitalopram** (Lexapro), **venlafaxine** (Effexor), and **paroxetine** (Paxil) appear less likely to inhibit CYP3A4 than fluvoxamine. **Fluoxetine** (Prozac) appears to be a weak inhibitor of CYP3A4, but little is known about the effect of other antidepressants on protease inhibitors.

- *Monitor*: If CYP3A4 inhibitors are used with these corticosteroids, monitor for evidence of corticosteroid toxicity such as hypertension, edema, diabetes, myopathy, ocular toxicity, and Cushing's syndrome (moon face, central obesity, bruising, hirsutism, acne).

OBJECT DRUGS	PRECIPITANT DRUGS	
Corticosteroids:	**Enzyme Inhibitors:**	
Budesonide (Entocort, Pulmicort)	**Amiodarone** (Cordarone)	**Diltiazem** (Cardizem)
	Amprenavir (Agenerase)	**Grapefruit**
Dexamethasone (Decadron)	**Aprepitant** (Emend)	**Indinavir** (Crixivan)
	Atazanavir (Reyataz)	**Nelfinavir** (Viracept)
Fluticasone (Flovent)	**Conivaptan** (Vaprisol)	**Ritonavir** (Norvir)
Methylprednisolone (Medrol)	**Cyclosporine** (Neoral)	**Saquinavir** (Invirase)
	Darunavir (Prezista)	**Verapamil** (Isoptin)
	Delavirdine (Rescriptor)	

COMMENTS: Inhibition of CYP3A4 may result in substantial increases in the plasma concentrations of these corticosteroids. This can lead to Cushing's syndrome and adrenal suppression. Although inhaled budesonide or fluticasone are not intended to act systemically, numerous cases have appeared of Cushing's syndrome and adrenal insufficiency due to concurrent use of potent CYP3A4.

CLASS 3: ASSESS RISK & TAKE ACTION IF NECESSARY

- *Consider Alternative*:

  Corticosteroids: Clinical evidence suggests that prednisone and prednisolone are less affected by CYP3A4 inhibitors, but one should still be alert for evidence of corticosteroid toxicity. Theoretically, beclomethasone is unlikely to be affected by CYP3A4 inhibitors.

  Calcium channel blockers: Calcium channel blockers other than diltiazem and verapamil are unlikely to inhibit CYP3A4.

  Grapefruit: Orange juice does not appear to inhibit CYP3A4.

- *Monitor*: If CYP3A4 inhibitors are used with these corticosteroids, monitor for evidence of corticosteroid toxicity such as hypertension, edema, diabetes, myopathy, ocular toxicity, and Cushing's syndrome (moon face, central obesity, bruising, hirsutism, acne).

-

OBJECT DRUGS	PRECIPITANT DRUGS	
Corticosteroids:	**Enzyme Inducers:**	
Betamethasone (Celestone)	**Barbiturates**	**Primidone** (Mysoline)
Cortisone (Cortone)	**Carbamazepine**	**Rifabutin**
Dexamethasone (Decadron)	(Tegretol)	(Mycobutin)
Hydrocortisone (Cortef)	**Efavirenz** (Sustiva)	**Rifampin** (Rifadin)
Methylprednisolone	**Nevirapine** (Viramune)	**Rifapentine** (Priftin)
(Medrol)	**Oxcarbazepine**	**St. John's Wort**
Prednisolone (Prelone)	(Trileptal)	**Topiramate**
Prednisone (Orasone)	**Phenytoin** (Dilantin)	(Topamax)
Triamcinolone (Aristocort)		

COMMENTS: Enzyme inducers can enhance the metabolism and reduce the therapeutic response to systemic corticosteroids. Increased corticosteroid dosage may be necessary. No adverse interaction would be expected if the corticosteroid is given topically or for other local effect, since reduced systemic exposure to the corticosteroid might actually reduce systemic adverse effects.

CLASS 3: ASSESS RISK & TAKE ACTION IF NECESSARY

- **Monitor:** Monitor the patient for reduced corticosteroid response if enzyme inducers are given concurrently. Substantial alterations in corticosteroid dosage may be necessary if enzyme inducers are initiated, discontinued, or changed in dosage. Keep in mind that enzyme induction is usually gradual and may take days to weeks for onset and offset, depending on the specific inducer.

OBJECT DRUGS	PRECIPITANT DRUGS
Digoxin (Lanoxin)	**Calcium Channel Blockers:**
	Bepridil (Vascor)
	Diltiazem (Cardizem)
	Verapamil (Isoptin)

COMMENTS: These calcium channel blockers inhibit P-glycoprotein and may reduce the renal and nonrenal elimination of digoxin. Digoxin plasma concentrations may increase substantially in some patients. Additive inhibition of A-V conduction may also occur. Nonetheless, with proper monitoring, digoxin is often used with these agents with good results.

CLASS 3: ASSESS RISK & TAKE ACTION IF NECESSARY

- **Consider Alternative:** Dihydropyridine calcium channel blockers such as **amlodipine** (Norvasc), **felodipine** (Plendil), or **nifedipine** (Procardia) do not appear to affect digoxin concentrations.
- **Monitor:** Monitor for altered digoxin effect if one of these calcium channel blockers is initiated, discontinued or changed in dosage; adjustments of digoxin dosage may be needed. Up to 10 days may be required for digoxin to achieve a new steady-state. If digoxin is initiated in the presence of therapy with one of these agents, consider conservative doses of digoxin.

OBJECT DRUGS	PRECIPITANT DRUGS	
Digoxin (Lanoxin)	**P-glycoprotein Inhibitors:**	
	Amiodarone (Cordarone)	**Nelfinavir** (Viracept)
	Azithromycin (Zithromax)	**Posaconazole** (Noxafil)
	Clarithromycin (Biaxin)	**Propafenone** (Rythmol)
	Conivaptan (Vaprisol)	**Quinidine** (Quinidex)
	Cyclosporine (Neoral)	**Ranolazine** (Ranexa)
	Dronedarone (Multaq)	**Ritonavir** (Norvir)
	Erythromycin (E-Mycin)	**Saquinavir** (Invirase)
	Hydroxychloroquine	**Tacrolimus** (Prograf)
	Indinavir (Crixivan)	**Telithromycin** (Ketek)
	Itraconazole (Sporanox)	**Tamoxifen** (Nolvadex)
	Ketoconazole (Nizoral)	

COMMENTS: Inhibitors of P-glycoprotein reduce the renal and nonrenal elimination of digoxin. Digoxin plasma concentrations may increase two- to four-fold but larger increases may occur especially with potent P-glycoprotein inhibitors such as quinidine or amiodarone. Clarithromycin appears to cause greater increases in digoxin plasma concentrations than erythromycin or azithromycin. The mechanism for the substantial increase in digoxin concentrations following concurrent use of hydroxychloroquine is not established. **Carvedilol** (Coreg) may produce small increases in digoxin plasma concentrations, although larger increases have been reported in children.

CLASS 3: ASSESS RISK & TAKE ACTION IF NECESSARY
- *Consider Alternative*:
  Macrolide Antibiotics: It is not known if dirithromycin* would interact with digoxin. (*not available in US)
- *Monitor*: Monitor for altered digoxin effect if one of these P-glycoprotein inhibitors is initiated, discontinued or changed in dosage; adjustments of digoxin dosage may be needed. Up to 10 days may be required for digoxin to achieve a new steady-state. If digoxin is initiated in the presence of therapy with one of these agents, consider conservative doses of digoxin.

OBJECT DRUGS		PRECIPITANT DRUGS	
Diuretics:		**Binding Resins:**	
Bumetanide (Bumex)	**Thiazides**	**Cholestyramine** (Questran)	
Furosemide (Lasix)	**Torsemide** (Demadex)	**Colestipol** (Colestid)	

COMMENTS: Cholestyramine and colestipol dramatically reduce furosemide and thiazide absorption and diuretic effect. The effect of binding resins on other diuretics is not established, but it may be prudent to take the same precautions with them as well. **Colesevelam** (Welchol) and **ezetimibe** (Zetia) appear less likely to bind with other drugs than cholestyramine and colestipol.

CLASS 3: ASSESS RISK & TAKE ACTION IF NECESSARY
- *Circumvent/Minimize*: Minimize the interaction by giving the diuretic 2 hours before or 6 hours after the binding resin; keep a constant interval between diuretic and binding resin.

- *Monitor*: Monitor for altered diuretic response if binding resins are initiated, discontinued, or dose is changed, or if the interval between doses of the diuretic and binding resin is changed.

OBJECT DRUGS	PRECIPITANT DRUGS
Dofetilide (Tikosyn)	**Inhibitors of Cationic Tubular Secretion:**
	Cimetidine (Tagamet)
	Ketoconazole (Nizoral)
	Triamterene (Dyrenium)
	Trimethoprim (Bactrim, Septra)

COMMENTS: Approximately 70% of dofetilide is renally eliminated unchanged via active cationic secretion and glomerular filtration. Dofetilide-induced QTc prolongation increases with increasing plasma concentrations. Any drug known to compete for cationic secretion could result in an increase in dofetilide plasma concentration. Pending more study, other drugs reported to inhibit cationic tubular secretion (e.g., **amiodarone**, **procainamide**, **diltiazem**, **metformin**, and **verapamil**) should be used only with careful monitoring in patients taking dofetilide. **Verapamil** and **ketoconazole** also may inhibit the CYP3A4 metabolism of dofetilide.

CLASS 3: ASSESS RISK & TAKE ACTION IF NECESSARY
- *Consider Alternative*:
  Cimetidine: Other H_2-receptor antagonists such as **famotidine** (Pepcid), **nizatidine** (Axid), and **ranitidine** (Zantac) could be used instead of cimetidine.
  Triamterene: **Spironolactone** (Aldactone) or **amiloride** (Midamor) could be used as a potassium-sparing diuretic.
- *Monitor*: Patients taking dofetilide should be carefully monitored for increased QTc intervals if drugs that reduce its renal clearance are coadministered.

OBJECT DRUGS	PRECIPITANT DRUGS
Dopamine Agonists:	**Dopamine Antagonists:**
Bromocriptine (Parlodel)	**Haloperidol** (Haldol)
Cabergoline (Dostinex)	**Metoclopramide** (Reglan)
Levodopa (Dopar)	**Phenothiazines**
Pramipexole (Mirapex)	**Thiothixene** (Navane)
Ropinirole (Requip)	

COMMENTS: Dopamine agonists, used for Parkinson's disease and other disorders, may be inhibited by dopamine antagonists resulting in a worsening of parkinsonism. Conversely, the therapeutic effect of dopamine antagonists would be expected to be reduced by dopamine agonists.

CLASS 2: USE ONLY IF BENEFIT FELT TO OUTWEIGH RISK
- *Use Alternative*:
  Antipsychotics: Atypical antipsychotics such as **clozapine** (Clozaril), **olanzapine** (Zyprexa), **quetiapine** (Seroquel), and **risperidone** (Risperdal) are less likely to produce extrapyramidal side effects. Theoretically, they would be

less likely than butyrophenones, phenothiazines, or thioxanthines to inhibit dopamine agonists.
- *Monitor*: Be alert for a reduction in efficacy of both dopamine agonists and dopamine antagonists if they are coadministered.

OBJECT DRUGS	PRECIPITANT DRUGS
Eplerenone (Inspra)	**Antimicrobials:**
	Clarithromycin (Biaxin)
	Erythromycin (E-Mycin)
	Fluconazole (Diflucan)
	Itraconazole (Sporanox)
	Ketoconazole (Nizoral)
	Posaconazole (Noxafil)
	Quinupristin (Synercid)
	Telithromycin (Ketek)
	Troleandomycin (TAO)
	Voriconazole (Vfend)

COMMENTS: Eplerenone is metabolized primarily by CYP3A4, and potent inhibitors of CYP3A4 may produce marked increases the serum levels of eplerenone. This may increase the risk of eplerenone toxicity, and the manufacturer states that eplerenone is contraindicated with potent CYP3A4 inhibitors.

CLASS 2: USE ONLY IF BENEFIT FELT TO OUTWEIGH RISK
- *Use Alternative*:
  Azole Antifungals: Itraconazole and ketoconazole are potent inhibitors of CYP3A4; fluconazole appears weaker, but in larger doses it also inhibits CYP3A4, and has been shown to produce moderate increases in plasma eplerenone concentrations.**Terbinafine** (Lamisil) does not appear to affect CYP3A4, and would not be expected to interact with eplerenone.
  Macrolide Antibiotics: Unlike erythromycin, clarithromycin and troleandomycin, **azithromycin** (Zithromax) and **dirithromycin*** do not appear to inhibit CYP3A4. (*not available in US)
  Telithromycin: The use of **azithromycin** (Zithromax) or a quinolone antibiotic should be considered.
- *Monitor*: If CYP3A4 inhibitors are used with eplerenone, monitor for excessive eplerenone effects such as hypotension and hyperkalemia; reduce eplerenone dose as needed.

OBJECT DRUGS	PRECIPITANT DRUGS
Eplerenone (Inspra)	**Antidepressants:**
	Fluvoxamine (Luvox)
	Nefazodone

COMMENTS: Eplerenone is metabolized primarily by CYP3A4, and potent inhibitors of CYP3A4 may produce marked increases the serum levels of eplerenone. This may increase the risk of eplerenone toxicity, and the manufacturer states that eplerenone is contraindicated with potent CYP3A4 inhibitors. Nefazodone is a potent CYP3A4 inhibitor, and fluvoxamine is a moderate inhibitor.

CLASS 2: USE ONLY IF BENEFIT FELT TO OUTWEIGH RISK
- *Use Alternative*: **Sertraline** (Zoloft), **citalopram** (Celexa), **escitalopram** (Lexapro), **venlafaxine** (Effexor), and **paroxetine** (Paxil) appear less likely to inhibit CYP3A4 than fluvoxamine. **Fluoxetine** (Prozac) appears to be a weak inhibitor of CYP3A4, but little is known about the effect of other antidepressants on eplerenone.
- *Monitor*: If CYP3A4 inhibitors are used with eplerenone, monitor for excessive eplerenone effects such as hypotension and hyperkalemia; reduce eplerenone dose as needed.

OBJECT DRUGS	PRECIPITANT DRUGS	
Eplerenone (Inspra)	**Enzyme Inhibitors:**	
	Amiodarone (Cordarone)	**Diltiazem** (Cardizem)
	Amprenavir (Agenerase)	**Grapefruit**
	Aprepitant (Emend)	**Indinavir** (Crixivan)
	Atazanavir (Reyataz)	**Nelfinavir** (Viracept)
	Conivaptan (Vaprisol)	**Ritonavir** (Norvir)
	Cyclosporine (Neoral)	**Saquinavir** (Invirase)
	Darunavir (Prezista)	**Verapamil** (Isoptin)
	Delavirdine (Rescriptor)	

COMMENTS: Eplerenone is metabolized primarily by CYP3A4, and inhibitors of CYP3A4 may produce marked increases the serum levels of eplerenone. This may increase the risk of eplerenone toxicity, and the manufacturer states that eplerenone is contraindicated with potent CYP3A4 inhibitors. Aprepitant is a moderate inhibitor of CYP3A4, but is also likely to increase eplerenone concentrations.

CLASS 2: USE ONLY IF BENEFIT FELT TO OUTWEIGH RISK
- *Use Alternative*: Use an alternative to the enzyme inhibitor if possible.
  Calcium channel blockers: Calcium channel blockers other than diltiazem and verapamil are unlikely to inhibit CYP3A4.
  Grapefruit: Orange juice does not appear to inhibit CYP3A4.
- *Monitor*: If CYP3A4 inhibitors are used with eplerenone, monitor for excessive eplerenone effects such as hypotension and hyperkalemia; reduce eplerenone dose as needed.

OBJECT DRUGS	PRECIPITANT DRUGS
Ergot Alkaloids:	**Antidepressants:**
Dihydroergotamine (D.H.E. 45)	**Fluvoxamine** (Luvox)
Ergotamine (Bellergal-S, Cafergot, Ergomar, Wigraine)	**Nefazodone**
Methysergide (Sansert)	

COMMENTS: Ergotamine (and probably dihydroergotamine and methysergide) undergo first-pass metabolism by CYP3A4, and several reports of ergotism have appeared when CYP3A4 inhibitors were given concurrently. Fluvoxamine appears to be a modest CYP3A4 inhibitor but may produce increased ergotamine concentrations. Theoretically non-oral routes of ergot administration would interact much less than the oral route.

CLASS 2: USE ONLY IF BENEFIT FELT TO OUTWEIGH RISK
- *Use Alternative*: **Sertraline** (Zoloft), **citalopram** (Celexa), **escitalopram** (Lexapro), **venlafaxine** (Effexor), and **paroxetine** (Paxil) appear less likely to inhibit CYP3A4 than fluvoxamine. **Fluoxetine** (Prozac) appears to be a weak inhibitor of CYP3A4. Little is known about the effects of other antidepressants on ergot alkaloids.
- *Monitor:* If the combination is used, monitor carefully for evidence of ergotism such as ischemia of extremities (pain, tenderness, cyanosis, and low skin temperature), hypertension, and tongue ischemia.

OBJECT DRUGS	PRECIPITANT DRUGS	
Ergot Alkaloids:	**Antimicrobials:**	
Dihydroergotamine	**Clarithromycin** (Biaxin)	**Posaconazole** (Noxafil)
(D.H.E. 45)	**Erythromycin** (E-Mycin)	**Quinupristin** (Synercid)
Ergotamine (Bellergal-S,	**Fluconazole** (Diflucan)	**Telithromycin** (Ketek)
Cafergot, Ergomar)	**Itraconazole** (Sporanox)	**Troleandomycin** (TAO)
Methysergide (Sansert)	**Ketoconazole** (Nizoral)	**Voriconazole** (Vfend)

COMMENTS: Ergotamine (and probably dihydroergotamine and methysergide) undergo first-pass metabolism by CYP3A4, and several reports of ergotism have appeared when CYP3A4 inhibitors were given concurrently. Theoretically non-oral routes of ergot administration would interact much less than the oral route.

CLASS 2: USE ONLY IF BENEFIT FELT TO OUTWEIGH RISK
- *Use Alternative*:
  Azole Antifungals: Itraconazole and ketoconazole are potent inhibitors of CYP3A4; fluconazole appears weaker, but in larger doses it also inhibits CYP3A4. **Terbinafine** (Lamisil) does not appear to affect CYP3A4, and would not be expected to interact with ergot alkaloids.
  Macrolide Antibiotics: Unlike erythromycin, clarithromycin and troleandomycin, **azithromycin** (Zithromax) and **dirithromycin*** do not appear to inhibit CYP3A4. (*not available in US)
  Telithromycin: The use of **azithromycin** (Zithromax) or a quinolone antibiotic should be considered.
- *Monitor*: If the combination is used, monitor carefully for evidence of ergotism such as ischemia of extremities (pain, tenderness, cyanosis, and low skin temperature), hypertension, and tongue ischemia.

OBJECT DRUGS	PRECIPITANT DRUGS	
Ergot Alkaloids:	**Enzyme Inhibitors:**	
Dihydroergotamine (D.H.E. 45)	**Amiodarone** (Cordarone)	**Imatinib** (Gleevec)
Ergotamine (Bellergal-S, Cafergot, Ergomar)	**Amprenavir** (Agenerase)	**Indinavir** (Crixivan)
Methysergide (Sansert)	**Aprepitant** (Emend)	**Lapatinib** (Tykerb)
	Atazanavir (Reyataz)	**Nelfinavir** (Viracept)
	Conivaptan (Vaprisol)	**Ritonavir** (Norvir)
	Cyclosporine (Neoral)	**Saquinavir** (Invirase)
	Darunavir (Prezista)	**Verapamil** (Isoptin)
	Delavirdine (Rescriptor)	
	Diltiazem (Cardizem)	
	Grapefruit	

COMMENTS: Ergotamine (and probably dihydroergotamine and methysergide) undergo first-pass metabolism by CYP3A4, and several reports of ergotism have appeared when CYP3A4 inhibitors were given concurrently. Theoretically non-oral routes of ergot administration would interact much less than the oral route. Some of these combinations are listed as contraindicated in the product information (e.g., amprenavir and ergot alkaloids).

CLASS 2: USE ONLY IF BENEFIT FELT TO OUTWEIGH RISK
- *Use Alternative:* If possible, select an alternative to the CYP3A4 inhibitor for patients receiving concomitant ergot alkaloids.
  Calcium channel blockers: Calcium channel blockers other than diltiazem and verapamil are unlikely to inhibit the metabolism of ergot alkaloids.
  Grapefruit: Orange juice does not appear to inhibit CYP3A4.
- *Monitor:* If the combination is used, monitor carefully for evidence of ergotism such as ischemia of extremities (pain, tenderness, cyanosis, and low skin temperature), hypertension, and tongue ischemia.

OBJECT DRUGS	PRECIPITANT DRUGS
Ergot Alkaloids:	**Triptans:**
Dihydroergotamine (D.H.E. 45)	**Almotriptan** (Axert)
Ergotamine (Bellergal-S, Cafergot, Ergomar, Wigraine)	**Eletriptan** (Relpax)
	Frovatriptan (Frova)
Methysergide (Sansert)	**Naratriptan** (Amerge)
	Rizatriptan (Maxalt)
	Sumatriptan (Imitrex)
	Zolmitriptan (Zolmig)

COMMENTS: Theoretically, concurrent use of ergot alkaloids and triptans may result in excessive vasoconstriction. The manufactures of triptans state that concurrent use with ergot preparations is contraindicated.

CLASS 1: AVOID COMBINATION
- *Avoid:* Avoid use of triptans within 24 hours of ergot alkaloids.

OBJECT DRUGS	PRECIPITANT DRUGS	
HMG-CoA Reductase	**Antimicrobials:**	
Inhibitors:	**Clarithromycin** (Biaxin)	**Posaconazole** (Noxafil)
Atorvastatin (Lipitor)	**Erythromycin** (E-Mycin)	**Quinupristin** (Synercid)
Lovastatin (Mevacor)	**Fluconazole** (Diflucan)	**Telithromycin** (Ketek)
Simvastatin (Zocor)	**Itraconazole** (Sporanox)	**Troleandomycin** (TAO)
	Ketoconazole (Nizoral)	**Voriconazole** (Vfend)

COMMENTS: Lovastatin and simvastatin undergo extensive first-pass metabolism by CYP3A4; antimicrobials that inhibit CYP3A4 increase the risk of myopathy, rhabdomyolysis and acute renal failure. Atorvastatin (Lipitor) undergoes less first-pass metabolism by CYP3A4 than lovastatin or simvastatin, so the risk of myopathy when combined with CYP3A4 inhibitors appears to be less. Nonetheless, some cases have been reported, including a fatal case of rhabdomyolysis possibly due to atorvastatin and fluconazole.

CLASS 2: USE ONLY IF BENEFIT FELT TO OUTWEIGH RISK
- *Use Alternative*:
  HMG-CoA Reductase Inhibitors: **Pravastatin** (Pravachol) is not metabolized by cytochrome P450 isozymes. **Fluvastatin** (Lescol) and **rosuvastatin** (Crestor) are metabolized by CYP2C9 and may interact with fluconazole and voriconazole.
  Azole Antifungals: Fluconazole appears to be a weaker inhibitor of CYP3A4 than itraconazole or ketoconazole. In larger doses it may inhibit CYP3A4 and should be used cautiously with lovastatin or simvastatin. Single doses of fluconazole would be unlikely to increase the risk of statin toxicity.
  Terbinafine (Lamisil) does not appear to inhibit CYP3A4.
  Macrolides: Unlike other macrolides, **azithromycin** (Zithromax) and **dirithromycin*** do not appear to inhibit CYP3A4 and would not be expected to interact with lovastatin or simvastatin. (*not available in US)
  Telithromycin: The use of **azithromycin** (Zithromax) or a quinolone antibiotic should be considered.
- *Circumvent/Minimize*: Discontinuation of the statin during antimicrobial treatment should be considered.
- *Monitor*: The patient should be alert for evidence of myopathy (muscle pain or weakness) and myoglobinuria (dark urine).

OBJECT DRUGS	PRECIPITANT DRUGS
HMG-CoA Reductase Inhibitors:	**Calcium Channel Blockers:**
Atorvastatin (Lipitor)	**Diltiazem** (Cardizem)
Lovastatin (Mevacor)	**Verapamil** (Isoptin)
Simvastatin (Zocor)	

COMMENTS: Lovastatin and simvastatin undergo extensive first-pass metabolism by CYP3A4; calcium channel blockers that inhibit CYP3A4 (diltiazem and verapamil) increase the statin serum concentrations, increasing the risk of myopathy, rhabdomyolysis and acute renal failure. Consider the increased risk of myopathy against the specific need for one of the calcium channel blockers that inhibits CYP3A4. Atorvastatin (Lipitor) undergoes less first-pass metabolism by

CYP3A4 than lovastatin or simvastatin, so the risk of myopathy when combined with CYP3A4 inhibitors appears to be less. Nonetheless, some cases have been reported.

CLASS 3: ASSESS RISK & TAKE ACTION IF NECESSARY

- **Consider Alternative**:
  HMG-CoA Reductase Inhibitors: **Pravastatin** (Pravachol) is not metabolized by cytochrome P450 isozymes, while **fluvastatin** (Lescol) and **rosuvastatin** (Crestor) are metabolized by CYP2C9—thus, they are not affected by CYP3A4 inhibition.
  Calcium channel blockers: Calcium channel blockers other than diltiazem and verapamil are unlikely to inhibit the metabolism of HMG-CoA reductase inhibitors.
- **Monitor**: If either diltiazem or verapamil is used with lovastatin or simvastatin, the patient should be alert for evidence of myopathy (muscle pain or weakness) and myoglobinuria (dark urine). Myopathy is usually associated with increased serum CK concentrations.

OBJECT DRUGS	PRECIPITANT DRUGS
HMG-CoA Reductase Inhibitors:	**Fibrates:**
Atorvastatin (Lipitor)	**Gemfibrozil** (Lopid)
Lovastatin (Mevacor)	
Rosuvastatin (Crestor)	
Simvastatin (Zocor)	

COMMENTS: Combined use of HMG-CoA reductase inhibitors and fibrates may increase the risk of myopathy, which may lead to rhabdomyolysis and acute renal failure. There appear to be differences in the relative risk, depending upon which HMG-CoA is used. Only rare cases of myopathy have been reported with atorvastatin and gemfibrozil, but the risk appears somewhat higher when lovastatin or simvastatin are coadministered with gemfibrozil. Gemfibrozil has been shown to substantially increase the serum concentrations of simvastatin acid and lovastatin acid. Gemfibrozil may produce moderate elevations of rosuvastatin plasma concentrations.

CLASS 3: ASSESS RISK & TAKE ACTION IF NECESSARY

- **Consider Alternative**:
  HMG-CoA Reductase Inhibitors: Although definitive incidence data are not available, the risk of myopathy during concurrent **pravastatin** (Pravachol) or **fluvastatin** (Lescol) with gemfibrozil or fenofibrate appears to be minimal.
  Gemfibrozil: The risk of myopathy with combined use of statins and fenofibrate appears to be less than with gemfibrozil. For example, fenofibrate does not appear to have a pharmacokinetic interaction with simvastatin.
- **Monitor**: If any HMG-CoA reductase inhibitor is used with gemfibrozil or another fibrate, the patient should be monitored for evidence of myopathy (muscle pain or weakness) and myoglobinuria (dark urine). Myopathy is usually associated with increased serum CK concentrations.

OBJECT DRUGS	PRECIPITANT DRUGS	
HMG-CoA Reductase Inhibitors: Atorvastatin (Lipitor) Lovastatin (Mevacor) Simvastatin (Zocor)	**Enzyme Inhibitors:** **Amiodarone** Cordarone) **Aprepitant** (Emend) **Amprenavir** (Agenerase) **Atazanavir** (Reyataz) **Conivaptan** (Vaprisol) **Cyclosporine** (Neoral) **Darunavir** (Prezista) **Delavirdine** (Rescriptor)	**Fluvoxamine** (Luvox) **Grapefruit** **Imatinib** (Gleevec) **Indinavir** (Crixivan) **Nefazodone** **Nelfinavir** (Viracept) **Ritonavir** (Norvir) **Saquinavir** (Invirase)

COMMENTS: Lovastatin and simvastatin undergo extensive first-pass metabolism by CYP3A4; inhibitors of CYP3A4 increase the risk of myopathy, in some cases leading to rhabdomyolysis and acute renal failure. Some of these combinations (e.g., atazanavir + lovastatin or simvastatin) are listed as contraindicated in the product information. Atorvastatin (Lipitor) undergoes less first-pass metabolism by CYP3A4 than lovastatin or simvastatin, so the risk of myopathy when combined with CYP3A4 inhibitors appears to be less. Nonetheless, some cases have been reported.

CLASS 2: USE ONLY IF BENEFIT FELT TO OUTWEIGH RISK

- *Use Alternative*:
  HMG-CoA Reductase Inhibitors: **Pravastatin** (Pravachol) is not metabolized by cytochrome P450 isozymes. **Fluvastatin** (Lescol), and **rosuvastatin** (Crestor) are metabolized by CYP2C9 and will not be affected by CYP3A4 inhibitors. [Note: Cyclosporine increases systemic exposure to *all* statins, although the risk of myopathy appears less with pravastatin.]
  Antidepressants: **Sertraline** (Zoloft), **citalopram** (Celexa), **venlafaxine** (Effexor), and **paroxetine** (Paxil) appear unlikely to inhibit CYP3A4, and **fluoxetine** (Prozac) appears to be a weak inhibitor of CYP3A4.
  Grapefruit: Orange juice does not appear to inhibit CYP3A4.
- *Monitor*: Patients receiving lovastatin or simvastatin and a CYP3A4 enzyme inhibitor should be the patient should be monitored for evidence of myopathy (muscle pain or weakness) and myoglobinuria (dark urine). Myopathy is usually associated with increased serum CK concentrations.

OBJECT DRUGS	PRECIPITANT DRUGS	
HMG-CoA Reductase Inhibitors: Atorvastatin (Lipitor) Lovastatin (Mevacor) Simvastatin (Zocor)	**Enzyme Inducers:** **Barbiturates** **Carbamazepine** (Tegretol) **Efavirenz** (Sustiva) **Etravirine** (Intelence) **Nevirapine** (Viramune) **Oxcarbazepine** (Trileptal)	**Phenytoin** (Dilantin) **Primidone** (Mysoline) **Rifabutin** (Mycobutin) **Rifampin** (Rifadin) **Rifapentine** (Priftin) **St. John's Wort**

COMMENTS: Atorvastatin, lovastatin, and simvastatin are metabolized CYP3A4 and enzyme inducers may substantially lower their serum concentrations. The magnitude of the effect may be sufficient to reduce the efficacy of the statin. For example, the potent inducer rifampin can lower simvastatin serum concentrations to less than 10% of normal, while even the modest enzyme inducer St. John's Wort can lower simvastatin serum concentrations to about one-third of normal. Although little is known about the effects of enzyme inducers on **fluvastatin** (Lescol), it is metabolized primarily by CYP2C9 and is likely to interact with enzyme inducers as well. **Rosuvastatin** (Crestor) has minimal CYP2C9 metabolism and will be unlikely to be affected by enzyme inducers.

CLASS 3: ASSESS RISK & TAKE ACTION IF NECESSARY

- *Consider Alternative*: If possible, select an alternative to the CYP3A4 inducer for patients receiving concomitant atorvastatin, lovastatin, or simvastatin. HMG-CoA Reductase Inhibitors: **Pravastatin** (Pravachol) is not metabolized by cytochrome P450 isozymes, and does not appear to be affected by enzyme inducers.

- *Monitor*: If atorvastatin, lovastatin, or simvastatin is used with an enzyme inducer, monitor for impairment of cholesterol-lowering effect. Keep in mind that enzyme induction is usually gradual and may take days to weeks for onset and offset, depending on the specific inducer.

OBJECT DRUGS	PRECIPITANT DRUGS	
Immunosuppressants:	**Enzyme Inducers:**	
Cyclosporine (Neoral)	**Barbiturates**	**Phenytoin** (Dilantin)
Sirolimus (Rapamune)	**Bosentan** (Tracleer)	**Primidone** (Mysoline)
Tacrolimus (Prograf)	**Carbamazepine** (Tegretol)	**Rifabutin** (Mycobutin)
	Efavirenz (Sustiva)	**Rifampin** (Rifadin)
	Levothyroxine (Synthroid)	**Rifapentine** (Priftin)
	Nevirapine (Viramune)	**St. John's Wort**
	Oxcarbazepine (Trileptal)	

COMMENTS: Enzyme inducers have been reported to enhance the metabolism of these immunosuppressants. This effect is probably due to induction of CYP3A4 and P-glycoprotein (PGP). Preliminary evidence suggests that levothyroxine acts as a PGP inducer in the small intestine; other thyroid hormones probably act similarly.

CLASS 2: USE ONLY IF BENEFIT FELT TO OUTWEIGH RISK

- *Use Alternative*: Use an alternative to the enzyme inducer if possible.

- *Monitor*: If an enzyme inducer is necessary, monitor for altered immunosuppressant effect if an enzyme inducer is initiated, discontinued, or changed in dosage; substantial dosage adjustments of immunosuppressants may be necessary. Keep in mind that enzyme induction is usually gradual and may take days to weeks for onset and offset, depending on the specific inducer.

OBJECT DRUGS	PRECIPITANT DRUGS	
Immunosuppressants:	**Antimicrobials:**	
Cyclosporine (Neoral)	**Azithromycin** (Zithromax)	**Ketoconazole** (Nizoral)
Sirolimus (Rapamune)	**Clarithromycin** (Biaxin)	**Posaconazole** (Noxafil)
Tacrolimus (Prograf)	**Clotrimazole** (Mycelex)	**Quinupristin** (Synercid)
	Erythromycin (E-Mycin)	**Telithromycin** (Ketek)
	Fluconazole (Diflucan)	**Troleandomycin** (TAO)
	Itraconazole (Sporanox)	**Voriconazole** (Vfend)

COMMENTS: These antimicrobial agents may inhibit the CYP3A4 metabolism of cyclosporine, sirolimus, and tacrolimus, thus increasing their effect and potential toxicity. Inhibition of P-glycoprotein (PGP) may also contribute to the interactions. Azithromycin does not inhibit CYP3A4, but appears to inhibit PGP; it may increase plasma concentrations of these immunosuppressants by this mechanism. Clotrimazole troches have been shown to elevate tacrolimus blood levels, and would also be expected to interact with cyclosporine and sirolimus. Some of these combinations are listed as contraindicated by the manufacturer (eg, sirolimus + voriconazole.)

CLASS 2: USE ONLY IF BENEFIT FELT TO OUTWEIGH RISK
- *Use Alternative*:
  Azole Antifungals: Itraconazole and ketoconazole are potent inhibitors of CYP3A4; fluconazole appears weaker, but in larger doses it also inhibits CYP3A4. **Terbinafine** (Lamisil) does not appear to affect CYP3A4, and would not be expected to interact with ergot alkaloids. In fact, terbinafine may slightly increase cyclosporine clearance according to the manufacturer.
  Macrolide Antibiotics: Consider using an alternative antibiotic.
  Telithromycin: Consider using an alternative antibiotic.
- *Monitor*: Monitor for altered immunosuppressant effect if a CYP3A4-inhibiting or PGP-inhibiting antimicrobial agent is initiated, discontinued, or changed in dosage.

OBJECT DRUGS	PRECIPITANT DRUGS	
Immunosuppressants:	**Enzyme Inhibitors:**	
Cyclosporine (Neoral)	**Amiodarone** (Cordarone)	**Diltiazem** (Cardizem)
Sirolimus (Rapamune)	**Amprenavir** (Agenerase)	**Fluvoxamine** (Luvox)
Tacrolimus (Prograf)	**Androgens**	**Grapefruit**
	Aprepitant (Emend)	**Indinavir** (Crixivan)
	Atazanavir (Reyataz)	**Methoxalen** (Oxsoralen)
	Chloroquine (Aralen)	**Nefazodone**
	Conivaptan (Vaprisol)	**Nelfinavir** (Viracept)
	Contraceptives, Oral	**Nicardipine** (Cardene)
	Danazol (Danocrine)	**Ritonavir** (Norvir)
	Darunavir (Prezista)	**Saquinavir** (Invirase)
	Delavirdine (Rescriptor)	**Verapamil** (Isoptin)

COMMENTS: The enzyme inhibitors listed here may inhibit cyclosporine, sirolimus, and tacrolimus elimination via CYP3A4 and/or P-glycoprotein (PGP), thus potentially increasing immunosuppressant effect and toxicity. Oral contraceptives also appear to increase cyclosporine plasma levels, although the mechanism is not clear. Aprepitant is a CYP3A4 inhibitor, but it had only a small effect on intravenous tacrolimus; oral tacrolimus would probably be more affected. Methoxalen produced modest increases in cyclosporine concentrations, but some subjects had substantial increases.

CLASS 2: USE ONLY IF BENEFIT FELT TO OUTWEIGH RISK

- *Use Alternative*: Use alternative to CYP3A4 inhibitor if possible.
  Antidepressants: **Sertraline** (Zoloft), **citalopram** (Celexa), **venlafaxine** (Effexor), and **paroxetine** (Paxil) appear less likely to inhibit CYP3A4 than fluvoxamine. **Fluoxetine** (Prozac) appears to be a weak inhibitor of CYP3A4.
  Calcium channel blockers: Calcium channel blockers other than diltiazem and verapamil are unlikely to inhibit CYP3A4.
  Grapefruit: Orange juice does not appear to inhibit CYP3A4.
- *Monitor*: If cyclosporine, sirolimus, or tacrolimus is initiated in the presence of CYP3A4 inhibitor therapy, it would be prudent to begin with conservative doses of the immunosuppressant. Monitor for altered immunosuppressant effect if an enzyme inhibitor is initiated, discontinued, or changed in dosage.

OBJECT DRUGS	PRECIPITANT DRUGS	
Lamotrigine (Lamictal)	**Enzyme Inducers:**	
	Barbiturates	**Primidone** (Mysoline)
	Carbamazepine (Tegretol)	**Rifabutin** (Mycobutin)
	Efavirenz (Sustiva)	**Rifampin** (Rifadin)
	Nevirapine (Viramune)	**Rifapentine** (Priftin)
	Oxcarbazepine (Trileptal)	**St. John's Wort**
	Phenytoin (Dilantin)	

COMMENTS: Enzyme-inducing drugs have been shown to reduce lamotrigine serum concentrations, probably by increasing lamotrigine glucuronidation. Some evidence suggests that lamotrigine may increase the risk of carbamazepine toxicity, but this has not been a consistent finding.

CLASS 3: ASSESS RISK & TAKE ACTION IF NECESSARY

- *Monitor*: Monitor for altered lamotrigine effect if enzyme inducers are initiated, discontinued, or changed in dosage. Adjustments in lamotrigine dosage may be necessary. Keep in mind that enzyme induction is usually gradual and may take days to weeks for onset and offset, depending on the specific inducer.

OBJECT DRUGS	PRECIPITANT DRUGS
Lamotrigine (Lamictal)	**Valproic Acid** (Depakene)

COMMENTS: Valproic acid may substantially increase lamotrigine serum concentrations, probably through inhibition of lamotrigine metabolism. It has also been proposed that the combination of lamotrigine and valproic acid may increase the risk of serious skin eruptions such as Stevens-Johnson syndrome or toxic epidermal necrolysis, but a causal relationship has not been established. Isolated cases of hyperammonemic encephalopathy have been reported in patients receiving lamotrigine and valproic acid concurrently, but more study is needed to establish the clinical importance.

CLASS 3: ASSESS RISK & TAKE ACTION IF NECESSARY

- *Monitor*: Monitor for altered lamotrigine effect if valproic acid is initiated, discontinued, or changed in dosage. Adjustments in lamotrigine dosage may be necessary. Monitor also for evidence of encephalopathy (lethargy, tremor, asterixis, and elevated ammonia levels).

OBJECT DRUGS	PRECIPITANT DRUGS
Lithium (Eskalith)	**Lithium Excretion Inhibitors:** **ACE Inhibitors** **Angiotensin Receptor Blockers (ARBs)** **COX-2 Inhibitors** **Loop Diuretics** **NSAIDs** **Thiazide Diuretics**

COMMENTS: Lithium toxicity has been reported when these agents are used with lithium, although the magnitude of the effect is highly variable from patient to patient. The elderly appear to be at greater risk. The lithium toxicity can be severe, and there are many case reports of lithium toxicity following initiation of one of these drugs. In an epidemiologic study ACE inhibitors and loop diuretics were associated with a substantial increase in the risk of hospitalization due to lithium toxicity, but an association with thiazide diuretics and NSAIDs was not found. It may be that only predisposed patients develop lithium toxicity from thiazides or NSAIDs; for example only some patients manifest substantial reductions in renal function following use of NSAIDs.

CLASS 3: ASSESS RISK & TAKE ACTION IF NECESSARY

- *Consider Alternative*:
  <u>ACE Inhibitors / Angiotensin Receptor Blockers</u>: An alternate agent such as a calcium channel blocker could be considered.
  <u>NSAIDs</u>: **Salicylates** do not appear to have much effect on plasma lithium concentrations and can be considered as alternatives to NSAIDs. **Sulindac** (Clinoril) appears less likely than other NSAIDs to increase lithium concentrations, but isolated cases have been reported. **Acetaminophen** is not likely to alter lithium elimination.
- *Monitor*: Monitor for altered lithium effects if these agents are initiated, discontinued, or changed in dosage. Note that—depending on the original lithium serum concentration—it may take up to several weeks for lithium toxicity to become manifest. Lithium toxicity may cause nausea, vomiting, anorexia, diarrhea, slurred speech, confusion, lethargy, coarse tremor, and in severe cases can cause seizures and coma.

OBJECT DRUGS	PRECIPITANT DRUGS
MAO Inhibitors (nonselective):	**Antidepressants, Tricyclic:**
Furazolidone (Furoxone)	**Clomipramine** (Anafranil)
Isocarboxazid	**Imipramine** (Tofranil)
Methylene Blue	
Phenelzine (Nardil)	
Tranylcypromine (Parnate)	

COMMENTS: Nonselective MAO inhibitors (MAOI) may produce serotonin syndrome when combined with tricyclic antidepressants (TCAs), especially TCAs with substantial serotonergic effects such as clomipramine and imipramine. Nonselective MAOI and TCAs have been used safely with careful monitoring in experienced hands, but serotonin syndrome can be life-threatening.

CLASS 1: AVOID COMBINATION
- *Avoid:* Avoid clomipramine and imipramine in patients receiving nonselective MAOI. Avoiding **amitriptyline, doxepin,** and **desipramine** would also be prudent although the risk is probably less. At least 14 days (preferably 18-20 days) should elapse after stopping an MAOI before starting clomipramine or imipramine. If a TCA is to be used, use those with less serotonergic effects and monitor for evidence of serotonin syndrome (myoclonus, rigidity, tremor, hyperreflexia, fever, sweating, seizures, confusion, agitation, incoordination, and coma).

OBJECT DRUGS	PRECIPITANT DRUGS	
MAO Inhibitors	**Serotonergic Drugs:**	
(nonselective):	**Buspirone** (BuSpar)	**Meperidine** (Demerol)
Furazolidone (Furoxone)	**Citalopram** (Celexa)	**Milnacipran** (Savella)
Isocarboxazid	**Cyclobenzaprine**	**Mirtazapine** (Remeron)
Methylene Blue	(Felxeril)	**Paroxetine** (Paxil)
Phenelzine (Nardil)	**Desvenlafaxine** (Pristiq)	**Propoxyphene** (Darvon)
Tranylcypromine (Parnate)	**Dextromethorphan**	**Sertraline** (Zoloft)
	Duloxetine (Cymbalta)	**Sibutramine** (Meridia)
	Escitalopram (Lexapro)	**Tetrabenazine**
	Fentanyl (Sublimaze)	(Xenazine)
	Fluoxetine (Prozac)	**Tramadol** (Ultram)
	Fluvoxamine (Luvox)	**Trazodone** (Desyrel)
		Venlafaxine (Effexor)

COMMENTS: Nonselective MAO inhibitors (MAOI) may produce serotonin syndrome when combined with serotonergic drugs. Serotonin syndrome can be life-threatening. (Note: Concurrent use of 2 or more serotonergic drugs (from the 2 right columns above) may increase the risk of serotonin syndrome, but only isolated cases have been reported.)

CLASS 1: AVOID COMBINATION
- *Avoid:* Avoid serotonergic drugs in patients receiving MAOI. At least 14 days (preferably 18-20 days) should elapse after stopping an MAOI before starting a

serotonergic drug. At least 5 weeks should elapse after stopping **fluoxetine** before starting an MAOI. If such combinations are used, monitor for evidence of serotonin syndrome (myoclonus, rigidity, tremor, hyperreflexia, fever, sweating, seizures, confusion, agitation, incoordination, and coma).

OBJECT DRUGS	PRECIPITANT DRUGS	
MAO Inhibitors **(nonselective):**	**Sympathomimetics:**	
Furazolidone (Furoxone)	**Amphetamines**	**Mazindol** (Sanorex)
	Atomoxetine (Strattera)	**Metaraminol** (Aramine)
Isocarboxazid	**Benzphetamine** (Didrex)	**Methamphetamine**
Methylene Blue	**Cocaine**	(Desoxyn)
Phenelzine (Nardil)	**Dextroamphetamine**	**Methylphenidate** (Ritalin)
Tranylcypromine (Parnate)	(Dexedrine)	**Phendimetrazine** (Bontril)
	Diethylpropion (Tenuate)	**Phentermine** (Ionamin)
	Dopamine	**Phenylephrine**
	Ephedrine	**Pseudoephedrine** (Sudafed)
	Isometheptene (Midrin)	**Tapentadol** (Nucynta)

COMMENTS: Indirect acting sympathomimetics and phenylephrine may result in severe hypertension, hyperpyrexia, seizures, arrhythmias and death in patients on nonselective MAO inhibitors (MAOI). Direct acting sympathomimetics such as **epinephrine**, **isoproterenol** and **norepinephrine** do not appear to interact as much, but one should still be alert for increased pressor effects.

CLASS 1: AVOID COMBINATION
- *Avoid:* Avoid the sympathomimetics for at least 14 days (preferably 18-20 days) after stopping an MAOI.

OBJECT DRUGS	PRECIPITANT DRUGS
MAO Inhibitors (nonselective):	**Antidepressants, Tricyclic:**
Linezolid (Zyvox)	**Clomipramine** (Anafranil)
	Imipramine (Tofranil)
MAO-B Inhibitors:	
Rasagiline (Azilect)	
Selegiline (Eldepryl)	

COMMENTS: Linezolid appears to be a weak MAOI, but serotonin syndrome has been reported when it is combined with serotonergic agents such as clomipramine and imipramine. Selective MAO-B inhibitors theoretically should not interact with TCAs, but in some patients MAO-B inhibitors may become nonselective thus increasing the risk of serotonin syndrome. Rasagiline is metabolized by CYP1A2, so theoretically, patients on CYP1A2 inhibitors may be more likely to develop nonselective MAO inhibition due to rasagiline. (For a list of CYP1A2 inhibitors, see CYP 450 Table at front of book.)

CLASS 2: USE ONLY IF BENEFIT FELT TO OUTWEIGH RISK
- *Use Alternative:* If a TCA is given to patients on linezolid or MAO-B inhibitors, use a TCA other than clomipramine or imipramine. Avoiding **amitriptyline**, **doxepin** and **desipramine** would also be prudent. The product

information for linezolid states that it should not be used with serotonergic agents unless the patient is closely observed for evidence of serotonin syndrome.
- *Monitor*: If any TCA is used with linezolid or an MAO-B inhibitor, monitor for evidence of serotonin syndrome (myoclonus, rigidity, tremor, hyperreflexia, fever, sweating, seizures, confusion, agitation, incoordination, and coma).

OBJECT DRUGS	PRECIPITANT DRUGS	
MAO Inhibitors (nonselective):	**Serotonergic Drugs:**	
Linezolid (Zyvox)	**Buspirone** (BuSpar)	**Milnacipran** (Savella)
	Citalopram (Celexa)	**Mirtazapine** (Remeron)
	Cyclobenzaprine (Felxeril)	**Paroxetine** (Paxil)
MAO-B Inhibitors:	**Desvenlafaxine** (Pristiq)	**Propoxyphene** (Darvon)
Rasagiline (Azilect)	**Dextromethorphan**	**Sertraline** (Zoloft)
Selegiline (Eldepryl)	**Duloxetine** (Cymbalta)	**Sibutramine** (Meridia)
	Escitalopram (Lexapro)	**Tetrabenazine** (Xenazine)
	Fentanyl (Sublimaze)	**Tramadol** (Ultram)
	Fluoxetine (Prozac)	**Trazodone** (Desyrel)
	Fluvoxamine (Luvox)	**Venlafaxine** (Effexor)
	Meperidine (Demerol)	

COMMENTS: Linezolid appears to be a weak MAOI, but serotonin syndrome has been reported when it is combined with serotonergic agents, including SSRIs and SNRIs. Selective MAO-B inhibitors theoretically should not interact with serotonergic drugs, and many patients have received these combinations safely. Some patients on MAO-B inhibitors, however, may develop nonselective MAO inhibition. Rasagiline is metabolized by CYP1A2, so theoretically, patients on CYP1A2 inhibitors may be more likely to develop nonselective MAO inhibition due to rasagiline. (For a list of CYP1A2 inhibitors, see CYP 450 Table at front of book.) (Note: Concurrent use of 2 or more serotonergic drugs (from the 2 right columns above) may increase the risk of serotonin syndrome, but only isolated cases have been reported.)

CLASS 2: USE ONLY IF BENEFIT FELT TO OUTWEIGH RISK
- *Use Alternative*: If possible use an alternative to the serotonergic drug in patients on linezolid or MAO-B inhibitors.
- *Monitor*: If serotonergic drugs are used with linezolid or MAO-B inhibitors, monitor for evidence of serotonin syndrome (myoclonus, rigidity, tremor, hyperreflexia, fever, sweating, seizures, confusion, agitation, incoordination, and coma).

OBJECT DRUGS	PRECIPITANT DRUGS	
MAO Inhibitors **(nonselective):**	**Sympathomimetics:**	
	Amphetamines	**Mazindol** (Sanorex)
Linezolid (Zyvox)	**Atomoxetine** (Strattera)	**Metaraminol** (Aramine)
	Benzphetamine (Didrex)	**Methamphetamine**
MAO-B Inhibitors:	**Cocaine**	(Desoxyn)
Rasagiline (Azilect)	**Dextroamphetamine**	**Methylphenidate** (Ritalin)
Selegiline (Eldepryl)	(Dexedrine)	**Phendimetrazine** (Bontril)
	Diethylpropion (Tenuate)	**Phentermine** (Ionamin)
	Dopamine	**Phenylephrine**
	Ephedrine	**Pseudoephedrine** (Sudafed)
	Isometheptene (Midrin)	**Tapentadol** (Nucynta)

COMMENTS: Linezolid is a mild MAO inhibitor, but can produce (usually modest) increases in the pressor response to indirect-acting sympathomimetics such as pseudoephedrine. MAO-B inhibitors theoretically would be unlikely to interact, but some patients on these drugs may develop nonselective MAO inhibition. Rasagiline is metabolized by CYP1A2, so theoretically, patients on CYP1A2 inhibitors may be more likely to develop nonselective MAO inhibition due to rasagiline. (For a list of CYP1A2 inhibitors, see CYP 450 Table at front of book.) Direct acting sympathomimetics such as **epinephrine**, **isoproterenol** and **norepinephrine** do not appear to interact as much with MAO inhibitors, but one should still be alert for increased pressor effects.

CLASS 2: USE ONLY IF BENEFIT FELT TO OUTWEIGH RISK
- *Monitor*: If sympathomimetic drugs are used with linezolid or MAO-B inhibitors, monitor for evidence of hypertension, fever, seizures, or arrhythmias; discontinue the sympathomimetics immediately if any of these findings are present.

OBJECT DRUGS	PRECIPITANT DRUGS	
Opioid Analgesics:	**Enzyme Inducers:**	
Alfentanil (Alfenta)	**Barbiturates**	
Codeine	**Bosentan** (Tracleer)	**Rifampin** (Rifadin)
Fentanyl (Sublimaze)	**Carbamazepine** (Tegretol)	**Rifapentine** (Priftin)
Methadone	**Efavirenz** (Sustiva)	**Ritonavir** (Norvir)
(Dolophine)	**Nevirapine** (Viramune)	**St. John's Wort**
Morphine	**Oxcarbazepine** (Trileptal)	
Oxycodone (Percocet)	**Phenytoin** (Dilantin)	
Sufentanil (Sufenta)	**Primidone** (Mysoline)	

COMMENTS: Enzyme inducers may increase the elimination of these opioids via CYP3A4 metabolism and possibly other pathways. This may result in reduced analgesic effects and may cause withdrawal symptoms in patients maintained on methadone. For example, rifampin has been shown to markedly reduce oxycodone plasma concentrations. Potent enzyme inducers such as rifampin may have larger effects on these analgesics than other inducers. With codeine, rifampin reduced the conversion of codeine to morphine, but only in those with normal CYP2D6 activity (EMs). Rifampin did not interact with codeine in subjects with little CYP2D6 activity (PMs), but PMs are not likely to have adequate analgesic effects from codeine whether or not they are taking enzyme inducers such as rifampin. Ritonavir may have variable effects on these opioids, depending on the duration of ritonavir therapy and other factors. In one study, ritonavir *increased* fentanyl plasma concentrations.

CLASS 3: ASSESS RISK & TAKE ACTION IF NECESSARY

- *Consider Alternative*: While it would be prudent to use an alternative to the enzyme inducer, suitable alternatives with equivalent therapeutic effects are not available for most enzyme inducers.
- *Monitor*: Monitor for reduced analgesic effect or evidence of methadone withdrawal (e.g., rhinorrhea, sweating, lacrimation, restlessness, and insomnia). Increase dose of opioid if needed. If the dose of the opioid is increased to compensate for the enzyme inducer, monitor for opioid toxicity if the enzyme inducer is stopped or reduced in dosage. Keep in mind that enzyme induction is usually gradual and may take days to weeks for onset and offset, depending on the specific inducer.

OBJECT DRUGS	PRECIPITANT DRUGS	
Opioid Analgesics:	**Antimicrobials:**	
Alfentanil (Alfenta)	**Clarithromycin** (Biaxin)	**Posaconazole** (Noxafil)
Fentanyl (Sublimaze)	**Clotrimazole** (Mycelex)	**Quinupristin** (Synercid)
Oxycodone (Percocet)	**Erythromycin** (E-Mycin)	**Telithromycin** (Ketek)
Sufentanil (Sufenta)	**Fluconazole** (Diflucan)	**Troleandomycin** (TAO)
	Itraconazole (Sporanox)	**Voriconazole** (Vfend)
	Ketoconazole (Nizoral)	

COMMENTS: These antimicrobials inhibit CYP3A4 and may inhibit the elimination of these opioids via CYP3A4 metabolism and possibly other pathways. Excessive opioid effects have been reported. For example, voriconazole produced almost a 4-fold increase in oxycodone plasma concentrations.

CLASS 3: ASSESS RISK & TAKE ACTION IF NECESSARY

- *Consider Alternative*:
  Azole Antifungals: Itraconazole and ketoconazole are potent inhibitors of CYP3A4; fluconazole appears weaker, but in larger doses it also inhibits CYP3A4. **Terbinafine** (Lamisil) does not appear to affect CYP3A4, and would not be expected to interact with ergot alkaloids. In fact, terbinafine may slightly increase cyclosporine clearance according to the manufacturer.
  Macrolide Antibiotics: Unlike erythromycin, clarithromycin and troleandomycin, **azithromycin** (Zithromax) and **dirithromycin*** do not appear to inhibit CYP3A4. (*not available in US)
  Telithromycin: The use of **azithromycin** (Zithromax) or a quinolone antibiotic should be considered.
- *Monitor*: Monitor for evidence of excessive and/or prolonged opioid effects, including sedation and respiratory depression.

OBJECT DRUGS	PRECIPITANT DRUGS	
Opioid Analgesics:	**Enzyme Inhibitors:**	
Alfentanil (Alfenta)	**Amiodarone** Cordarone)	**Diltiazem** (Cardizem)
Fentanyl (Sublimaze)	**Amprenavir** (Agenerase)	**Fluvoxamine** (Luvox)
Oxycodone (Percocet)	**Aprepitant** (Emend)	**Grapefruit**
Sufentanil (Sufenta)	**Atazanavir** (Reyataz)	**Indinavir** (Crixivan)
	Cimetidine (Tagamet)	**Nefazodone**
	Conivaptan (Vaprisol)	**Nelfinavir** (Viracept)
	Cyclosporine (Neoral)	**Ritonavir** (Norvir)
	Darunavir (Prezista)	**Saquinavir** (Invirase)
	Delavirdine (Rescriptor)	**Verapamil** (Isoptin)

COMMENTS: These enzyme inhibitors may inhibit the elimination of these opioids via CYP3A4 metabolism and possibly other pathways. Excessive opioid effects have been reported. The magnitude of the interaction may vary considerably depending on the inhibitor. Some inhibitors (e.g., cyclosporine, nefazodone) are more potent than weaker inhibitors such as cimetidine. Nonetheless, cimetidine produced a large increase in alfentanil half-life and large reduction in alfentanil clearance.

CLASS 3: ASSESS RISK & TAKE ACTION IF NECESSARY

- *Consider Alternative*:
  Calcium channel blockers: Calcium channel blockers other than diltiazem and verapamil are unlikely to inhibit CYP3A4.
  Cimetidine: **Famotidine** (Pepcid), **nizatidine** (Axid), and **ranitidine** (Zantac) have minimal effects on drug metabolism. In one study, ranitidine had no effect on alfentanil pharmacokinetics.
  Grapefruit: Orange juice does not appear to inhibit CYP3A4.
  Antidepressants: **Sertraline** (Zoloft), **citalopram** (Celexa), **venlafaxine** (Effexor), and **paroxetine** (Paxil) appear less likely to inhibit CYP3A4 than fluvoxamine, and much less likely than nefazodone. **Fluoxetine** (Prozac) appears to be a weak inhibitor of CYP3A4.
- *Monitor*: Monitor for evidence of excessive and/or prolonged opioid effects, including sedation and respiratory depression.

OBJECT DRUGS	PRECIPITANT DRUGS	
Opioid Analgesics	**SSRI and SNRI:**	
(Serotonergic):	**Citalopram** (Celexa)	**Fluvoxamine** (Luvox)
Alfentanil (Alfenta)	**Clomipramine** (Anafranil)	**Imipramine** (Tofranil)
Fentanyl (Sublimaze)	**Desvenlafaxine** (Pristiq)	**Milnacipran** (Savella)
Meperidine (Demerol)	**Duloxetine** (Cymbalta)	**Paroxetine** (Paxil)
Tramadol (Ultram)	**Escitalopram** (Lexapro)	**Sertraline** (Zoloft)
	Fluoxetine (Prozac)	**Venlafaxine** (Effexor)

COMMENTS: There have been a number of cases of serotonin syndrome following the combined used of serotonergic analgesics such as meperidine or tramadol with selective serotonin reuptake inhibitors (SSRI) or selective serotonin-norepinephrine reuptake inhibitors (SNRI). One case of fatal serotonin syndrome was reported in a patient on **amitriptyline** following the addition of tramadol. Limited evidence suggests that **fentanyl** may also exhibit additive serotonergic effects with other serotonergic drugs, but more evidence is needed.

CLASS 3: ASSESS RISK & TAKE ACTION IF NECESSARY

- *Consider Alternative*:
  Opioid Analgesic: In patients taking an SSRI or SNRI consider using an alternative to meperidine or tramadol.
  Antidepressant: If a tricyclic antidepressant (TCA) is given to patients on meperidine or tramadol, use a TCA other than clomipramine or imipramine. Avoiding **amitriptyline**, **doxepin** and **desipramine** would also be prudent.
- *Monitor*: If the combination is used monitor for evidence of serotonin syndrome (myoclonus, rigidity, tremor, fever, sweating, seizures, confusion, agitation, incoordination, and coma).

OBJECT DRUGS	PRECIPITANT DRUGS	
Methotrexate (Antineoplastic Doses)	**Inhibitors of Anionic Tubular Secretion:**	
	Aspirin	**Pantoprazole** (Protonix)
Pralatrexate (Folotyn)	**Ciprofloxacin** (Cipro)	**Penicillins**
	Co-trimoxazole (Septra)	**Probenecid** (Benemid)
	NSAIDs	**Salicylates**
	Omeprazole (Prilosec)	**Thiazide**

COMMENTS: In patients receiving antineoplastic doses of methotrexate, ciprofloxacin, NSAIDs, penicillins (e.g., amoxicillin, carbenicillin, mezlocillin, oxacillin, piperacillin, etc.) and salicylates have been associated with methotrexate toxicity such as bone marrow suppression and GI toxicity. Little is known regarding the effect of other proton pump inhibitors on methotrexate. A causal relationship is not well established, but the severity of the reactions dictates caution. The risk with low-dose methotrexate (e.g., for arthritis) is probably much lower; indeed, NSAIDs are often used with low-dose methotrexate in the situation. Nonetheless, one should still be alert for evidence of methotrexate toxicity. Probenecid can increase methotrexate levels by 2-3 fold. The effect of quinolones other than ciprofloxacin on methotrexate is not established, but be alert for evidence of methotrexate toxicity. Pralatrexate concentrations are increased by probenecid; caution with other inhibitors of renal clearance is warranted.

CLASS 2: USE ONLY IF BENEFIT FELT TO OUTWEIGH RISK

- *Use Alternative*:
  Salicylates or NSAIDs: Consider **acetaminophen** instead of salicylates or NSAIDs. Preliminary evidence suggests that **celecoxib** (Celebrex) does not affect methotrexate pharmacokinetics and could be considered as an alternative. **Valdecoxib** (withdrawn from US market), however, may increase methotrexate serum concentrations.
- *Monitor*: Monitor for altered dihydrofolate reductase inhibitor effect if a renal tubular secretion inhibitor is initiated, discontinued, or changed in dose.

OBJECT DRUGS	PRECIPITANT DRUGS
Mycophenolate (CellCept)	**Binding Agents:**
	Antacids
	Calcium Polycarbophil (FiberCon, Konsyl)
	Cholestyramine (Questran)
	Colestipol (Colestid)
	Iron
	Sucralfate (Carafate)

COMMENTS: Cholestyramine can substantially reduce mycophenolate mofetil (MM) serum concentrations by binding in the gastrointestinal tract and interfering with its enterohepatic circulation. Colestipol theoretically would have a similar effect. Aluminum-magnesium antacids modestly reduce MM absorption. The affect of iron on MM may be less in patients taking cyclosporine plus MM.

CLASS 3: ASSESS RISK & TAKE ACTION IF NECESSARY
- *Circumvent/Minimize*: Since the interaction appears to be due to interruption of MM enterohepatic circulation, separation of doses is not likely to circumvent the interaction completely. Nonetheless, if the combination is used, separate the doses as much as possible and monitor for reduced MM effect.
- *Consider Alternative*:
  Lipid Lowering Agents: The use of alternative hypolipidemic such as HMG-CoA reductase inhibitors should be considered. **Colesevelam** (Welchol) and **ezetimibe** (Zetia) appear less likely to bind with drugs than cholestyramine and colestipol.
  Antacids: Antisecretory agents such as H_2-receptor antagonists or proton pump inhibitors would be less likely to interact than antacids.
- *Monitor*: Patients receiving mycophenolate with binding resins or antacids should be monitored for reduced immunosuppressant efficacy.

OBJECT DRUGS	PRECIPITANT DRUGS
Nitrates:	**Sildenafil** (Viagra)
Isosorbide Dinitrate (Isordil)	**Tadalafil** (Cialis)
Isosorbide Mononitrate (Ismo)	**Vardenafil** (Levitra)
Nitroglycerin (Nitrogard)	

COMMENTS: Sildenafil, tadalafil, and vardenafil may markedly enhance the hypotensive effects of nitrates. Fatalities have been reported, although a causal relationship was not established in some cases. Other vasodilators such as **terazosin** (Hytrin) and **doxazosin** (Cardura) have also been reported to produce hypotensive episodes when coadministered with phosphodiesterase inhibitors.

CLASS 1: AVOID COMBINATION
- *Avoid*: Patients taking nitrates by any route of administration should avoid taking phosphodiesterase inhibitors.

OBJECT DRUGS		PRECIPITANT DRUGS
NSAIDs:		**SSRI and SNRI:**
Diclofenac (Voltaren)	**Mefenamic acid**	**Citalopram** (Celexa)
Diflunisal (Dolobid)	**Meloxicam** (Mobic)	**Clomipramine** (Anafranil)
Etodolac (Lodine)	**Nabumetone** (Relafen)	**Desvenlafaxine** (Pristiq)
Fenoprofen (Nalfon)	**Naproxen** (Aleve)	**Duloxetine** (Cymbalta)
Flurbiprofen (Ansaid)	**Oxaprozin** (Daypro)	**Escitalopram** (Lexapro)
Ibuprofen (Motrin)	**Piroxicam** (Feldene)	**Fluoxetine** (Prozac)
Indomethacin	**Sulindac** (Clinoril)	**Fluvoxamine** (Luvox)
(Indocin)	**Tolmetin** (Tolectin)	**Imipramine** (Tofranil)
Ketoprofen (Orudis)		**Milnacipran** (Savella)
Ketorolac (Toradol)		**Paroxetine** (Paxil)
Meclofenamate		**Sertraline** (Zoloft)
		Venlafaxine (Effexor)

COMMENTS: Some studies suggest that the concurrent use of NSAIDs or aspirin with serotonin reuptake inhibitors (SSRI) or serotonin-norepinephrine uptake inhibitors (SNRI) increases the risk of gastrointestinal (GI) bleeding compared to either drug used alone. Some evidence suggests that even low-dose aspirin may increase GI bleeding when combined with SSRIs or SNRIs. However, the vast majority of patients on concurrent therapy with an NSAID or aspirin and an SSRI will not develop GI bleeding. Since GI bleeding can be fatal, however, anything that increases the risk should be avoided if possible. The putative mechanism is inhibition of serotonin uptake by platelets added to gastric toxicity and antiplatelet effect caused by the NSAIDs. The risk of GI bleeding appears to be related to the potency of the serotonin reuptake inhibition, a finding that lends additional support to the existence of an interaction.

CLASS 3: ASSESS RISK & TAKE ACTION IF NECESSARY

• *Consider Alternative*:
  NSAIDs: If the NSAID is being used as an analgesic, consider using acetaminophen instead. COX-2 inhibitors do not affect platelets, and may offer a lower risk of GI bleeding when combined with a SSRI.
  Antidepressant: If appropriate for the patient, consider using agents with low serotonin reuptake inhibition such as **desipramine** (Norpramin), **maprotiline** (Ludiomil), **nortriptyline** (Aventyl), **trimipramine** (Surmontil) or moderate serotonin reuptake inhibitors such as **amitriptyline** (Elavil) or **imipramine** (Tofranil)

• *Monitor*: Patients and health professionals should be alert for evidence of gastrointestinal bleeding if these combinations are used.

OBJECT DRUGS	PRECIPITANT DRUGS	
Fosphenytoin (Cerebyx) **Phenytoin** (Dilantin)	**Enzyme Inhibitors:**	
	Amiodarone (Cordarone)	**Fluorouracil** (5-FU)
	Androgens	**Fluoxetine** (Prozac)
	Capecitabine (Xeloda)	**Fluvoxamine** (Luvox)
	Chloramphenicol	**Imatinib** (Gleevec)
	Cimetidine (Tagamet)	**Isoniazid** (INH)
	Co-trimoxazole (Bactrim)	**Leflunomide** (Arava)
	Danazol (Danocrine)	**Metronidazole** (Flagyl)
	Delavirdine (Rescriptor)	**Sulfinpyrazone** (Anturane)
	Disulfiram (Antabuse)	**Tamoxifen** (Nolvadex)
	Efavirenz (Sustiva)	**Ticlopidine** (Ticlid)
	Fluconazole (Diflucan)	**Voriconazole** (Vfend)

COMMENTS: Inhibitors of CYP2C9 (and to a lesser extent CYP2C19) may increase phenytoin levels; phenytoin toxicity may occur. Depending on the baseline phenytoin serum concentration, it may take as long as several weeks for phenytoin toxicity to occur after starting an inhibitor.

CLASS 3: ASSESS RISK & TAKE ACTION IF NECESSARY

- *Consider Alternative*:

  Azole Antifungals: **Ketoconazole** (Nizoral) and **itraconazole** (Sporanox) appear to be less likely to affect phenytoin.

  Cimetidine: **Famotidine** (Pepcid), **nizatidine** (Axid), and **ranitidine** (Zantac) have minimal effects on drug metabolism.

  Fluvastatin: HMG-CoA reductase inhibitors other than fluvastatin do not appear to inhibit CYP2C9.

  SSRIs: The use of SSRIs that do not inhibit CYP2C9 [eg, **paroxetine** (Paxil) or **venlafaxine** (Effexor)] should be considered.

- *Monitor*: Monitor for altered phenytoin effect if an inhibitor is initiated, discontinued, or changed in dosage. Evidence of phenytoin toxicity includes nystagmus, ataxia, diplopia, drowsiness, and lethargy; severe cases may result in asterixis and coma.

OBJECT DRUGS	PRECIPITANT DRUGS	
Pimozide (Orap)	**Antimicrobials:**	
	Clarithromycin (Biaxin)	**Posaconazole** (Noxafil)
	Erythromycin (E-Mycin)	**Quinupristin** (Synercid)
	Fluconazole (Diflucan)	**Telithromycin** (Ketek)
	Itraconazole (Sporanox)	**Troleandomycin** (TAO)
	Ketoconazole (Nizoral)	**Voriconazole** (Vfend)

COMMENTS: Pimozide alone can prolong the QT interval, and it has been associated with ventricular arrhythmias (torsades de pointes). Drugs that inhibit CYP3A4 may increase pimozide serum concentrations.

CLASS 1: AVOID COMBINATION

- **Avoid**: These antimicrobials should not be given to patients receiving pimozide due to the risk of life-threatening ventricular arrhythmias.
- **Use Alternative**:

  Azole Antifungals: Itraconazole and ketoconazole are potent inhibitors of CYP3A4: fluconazole appears weaker, but in larger doses it also inhibits CYP3A4. **Terbinafine** (Lamisil) does not appear to affect CYP3A4, and would not be expected to interact with pimozide.

  Macrolide Antibiotics: Unlike erythromycin, clarithromycin and troleandomycin, **azithromycin** (Zithromax) and **dirithromycin*** do not appear to inhibit CYP3A4. (*not available in US)

  Telithromycin: The use of **azithromycin** (Zithromax) or a quinolone antibiotic should be considered.

OBJECT DRUGS	PRECIPITANT DRUGS	
Pimozide (Orap)	**Enzyme Inhibitors:**	
	Amiodarone (Cordarone)	**Grapefruit**
	Amprenavir (Agenerase)	**Indinavir** (Crixivan)
	Aprepitant (Emend)	**Nefazodone**
	Atazanavir (Reyataz)	**Nelfinavir** (Viracept)
	Conivaptan (Vaprisol)	**Paroxetine** (Paxil)
	Cyclosporine (Neoral)	**Ritonavir** (Norvir)
	Darunavir (Prezista)	**Saquinavir** (Invirase)
	Delavirdine (Rescriptor)	**Sertraline** (Zoloft)
	Diltiazem (Cardizem)	**Verapamil** (Isoptin)
	Fluvoxamine (Luvox)	

COMMENTS: Pimozide alone can prolong the QT interval, and it has been associated with ventricular arrhythmias (torsades de pointes). Drugs that inhibit CYP3A4 may increase pimozide serum concentrations and increase the risk of ventricular arrhythmias. Orap product information states that pimozide is contraindicated with indinavir, nelfinavir, ritonavir, saquinavir, and other CYP3A4 inhibitors. The mechanism for increased pimozide serum concentrations with **paroxetine** and **sertraline** is not known, but the product information contraindicates the combinations.

CLASS 1: AVOID COMBINATION

- **Avoid**: CYP3A4 inhibitors should not be given to patients receiving pimozide due to the risk of life-threatening ventricular arrhythmias. Use an alternative drug to the CYP3A4 inhibitor if possible.
- **Use Alternative**:

  Antidepressants: **Citalopram** (Celexa), **venlafaxine** (Effexor), and **paroxetine** (Paxil) appear less likely to inhibit CYP3A4 than fluvoxamine. **Fluoxetine** (Prozac) appears to be a weak inhibitor of CYP3A4.

  Calcium channel blockers: Calcium channel blockers other than diltiazem and verapamil are unlikely to inhibit CYP3A4.

  Grapefruit: Orange juice does not appear to inhibit CYP3A4.

OBJECT DRUGS	PRECIPITANT DRUGS
Drugs Increasing Potassium:	**Drugs Increasing Potassium:**
ACE inhibitors	**ACE inhibitors**
Potassium-sparing diuretics	**Potassium-sparing diuretics**
Potassium supplements	**Potassium supplements**

COMMENTS: Concurrent use of more than one agent that increases serum potassium may lead to additive hyperkalemic effects and excessive serum potassium levels, especially in the presence of one or more predisposing factors such as significant renal impairment, severe diabetes, high potassium diet, and advanced age. Fatal hyperkalemia has occurred, but is rare. ACE inhibitors are frequently used with potassium-sparing diuretics with good results, but close monitoring is necessary in patients with risk factors. Other drugs that may exhibit hyperkalemic activity include **drospirenone** (Yasmin), **heparins, nonselective beta-blockers, NSAIDs, COX-2 inhibitors, angiotensin receptor antagonists, cyclosporine, tacrolimus, succinylcholine, pentamidine, trimethoprim**, and **potassium-containing salt substitutes**.

CLASS 3: ASSESS RISK & TAKE ACTION IF NECESSARY
- *Monitor:* Monitor serum potassium concentrations, especially in patients with predisposing factors such as renal disease, diabetes, and advanced age.

OBJECT DRUGS	PRECIPITANT DRUGS
Procainamide (Pronestyl)	**Cimetidine** (Tagamet)
	Co-trimoxazole (Bactrim, Septra)
	Ketoconazole (Nizoral)
	Levofloxacin (Levaquin)
	Triamterene (Dyrenium)

COMMENTS: The renal clearance of procainamide may be reduced by these drugs, resulting in elevated procainamide concentrations, particularly in patients with renal dysfunction. Pending more study, other drugs reported to inhibit cationic tubular secretion (e.g., **amiodarone, dofetilide, diltiazem, metformin**, and **verapamil**) should be used with careful monitoring in patients taking procainamide.

CLASS 3: ASSESS RISK & TAKE ACTION IF NECESSARY
- *Consider Alternative:*
  Cimetidine: Other H_2-receptor antagonists such as **famotidine** (Pepcid), **nizatidine** (Axid), and **ranitidine** (Zantac) could be used instead of cimetidine.
  Triamterene: **Spironolactone** (Aldactone) or **amiloride** (Midamor) could be used as a potassium-sparing diuretic.
- *Monitor:* Be alert for increased procainamide effects (e.g., prolonged QRS or QTc intervals) in patients taking drugs that are known to reduce cationic renal clearance.

OBJECT DRUGS	PRECIPITANT DRUGS
Protease Inhibitors:	**Enzyme Inducers:**
Amprenavir (Agenerase)	**Barbiturates**
Atazanavir (Reyataz)	**Bosentan** (Tracleer)
Darunavir (Prezista)	**Carbamazepine** (Tegretol)
Delavirdine (Rescriptor)	**Efavirenz** (Sustiva)
Fosamprenavir (Lexiva)	**Nevirapine** (Viramune)
Indinavir (Crixivan)	**Oxcarbazepine** (Trileptal)
Lopinavir (Kaletra)	**Phenytoin** (Dilantin)
Nelfinavir (Viracept)	**Primidone** (Mysoline)
Ritonavir (Norvir)	**Rifabutin** (Mycobutin)
Saquinavir (Invirase)	**Rifampin** (Rifadin)
Tipranavir (Aptivus)	**Rifapentine** (Priftin)
	St. John's Wort

COMMENTS: Enzyme inducers may reduce the serum levels of the protease inhibitors resulting in loss of efficacy or emergence of resistant viral strains. Some combinations result in dramatic reductions in protease inhibitor serum concentrations (e.g., delavirdine + rifampin, and atazanavir + rifampin). The combination of ritonavir and rifabutin may increase the risk of rifabutin uveitis (See Rifabutin + Enzyme Inhibitors).

CLASS 3: ASSESS RISK & TAKE ACTION IF NECESSARY

- *Consider Alternative*: Use an alternative to the enzyme inducer if possible. Rifampin is particularly problematic, since it can produce dramatic reductions in the plasma concentrations of protease inhibitors.
- *Circumvent/Minimize*: Consider increasing the dose of the protease inhibitor if enzyme inducers are coadministered.
- *Monitor*: If it is necessary to use protease inhibitors and enzyme inducers monitor for loss of anti-viral efficacy. Keep in mind that enzyme induction is usually gradual and may take days to weeks for onset and offset, depending on the specific inducer.

OBJECT DRUGS	PRECIPITANT DRUGS
Protease Inhibitors:	**Antimicrobials:**
Amprenavir (Agenerase)	**Clarithromycin** (Biaxin)
Atazanavir (Reyataz)	**Erythromycin** (E-Mycin)
Darunavir (Prezista)	**Fluconazole** (Diflucan)
Delavirdine (Rescriptor)	**Itraconazole** (Sporanox)
Fosamprenavir (Lexiva)	**Ketoconazole** (Nizoral)
Indinavir (Crixivan)	**Posaconazole** (Noxafil)
Lopinavir (Kaletra)	**Quinupristin** (Synercid)
Nelfinavir (Viracept)	**Telithromycin** (Ketek)
Ritonavir (Norvir)	**Troleandomycin** (TAO)
Saquinavir (Invirase)	**Voriconazole** (Vfend)
Tipranavir (Aptivus)	

COMMENTS: Inhibitors of CYP3A4 may increase the serum levels of the protease inhibitors resulting in increased side effects. **Ritonavir** may substantially increase **voriconazole** plasma concentrations, especially in patients deficient in CYP2C19.

CLASS 3: ASSESS RISK & TAKE ACTION IF NECESSARY

- *Consider Alternative*:
  Azole Antifungals: Itraconazole and ketoconazole are potent inhibitors of CYP3A4; fluconazole appears weaker, but in larger doses it also inhibits CYP3A4. **Terbinafine** (Lamisil) does not appear to affect CYP3A4, and would not be expected to interact with protease inhibitors.
  Macrolide Antibiotics: Unlike erythromycin, clarithromycin and troleandomycin, **azithromycin** (Zithromax) and **dirithromycin*** do not appear to inhibit CYP3A4. (*not available in US)
  Telithromycin: The use of **azithromycin** (Zithromax) or a quinolone antibiotic should be considered.
- *Circumvent/Minimize*: Consider reducing the dose of the protease inhibitor if enzyme inhibitors are coadministered.
- *Monitor*: Monitor for protease inhibitor toxicity.

OBJECT DRUGS		PRECIPITANT DRUGS
Protease Inhibitors:		**Antidepressants:**
Amprenavir (Agenerase)	**Lopinavir** (Kaletra)	**Fluvoxamine** (Luvox)
Atazanavir (Reyataz)	**Nelfinavir** (Viracept)	**Nefazodone**
Darunavir (Prezista)	**Ritonavir** (Norvir)	
Delavirdine (Rescriptor)	**Saquinavir** (Invirase)	
Fosamprenavir (Lexiva)	**Tipranavir** (Aptivus)	
Indinavir (Crixivan)		

COMMENTS: Inhibitors of CYP3A4 may increase the serum levels of the protease inhibitors resulting in increased side effects.

CLASS 3: ASSESS RISK & TAKE ACTION IF NECESSARY

- *Consider Alternative*: **Sertraline** (Zoloft), **citalopram** (Celexa), **escitalopram** (Lexapro), **venlafaxine** (Effexor), and **paroxetine** (Paxil) appear less likely to inhibit CYP3A4 than fluvoxamine. **Fluoxetine** (Prozac) appears to be a weak inhibitor of CYP3A4, but little is known about the effect of other antidepressants on protease inhibitors.
- *Circumvent/Minimize*: Consider reducing the dose of the protease inhibitor if enzyme inhibitors are coadministered.
- *Monitor*: Monitor for protease inhibitor toxicity.

OBJECT DRUGS	PRECIPITANT DRUGS
Protease Inhibitors:	**Enzyme Inhibitors:**
Amprenavir (Agenerase)	**Amiodarone** (Cordarone)
Atazanavir (Reyataz)	**Amprenavir** (Agenerase)
Darunavir (Prezista)	**Aprepitant** (Emend)
Delavirdine (Rescriptor)	**Atazanavir** (Reyataz)
Fosamprenavir (Lexiva)	**Conivaptan** (Vaprisol)
Indinavir (Crixivan)	**Cyclosporine** (Neoral)
Lopinavir (Kaletra)	**Darunavir** (Prezista)
Nelfinavir (Viracept)	**Delavirdine** (Rescriptor)
Ritonavir (Norvir)	**Diltiazem** (Cardizem)
Saquinavir (Invirase)	**Grapefruit**
Tipranavir (Aptivus)	**Indinavir** (Crixivan)
	Nelfinavir (Viracept)
	Ritonavir (Norvir)
	Saquinavir (Invirase)
	Verapamil (Isoptin)

COMMENTS: Inhibitors of CYP3A4 may increase the serum levels of the protease inhibitors resulting in increased side effects.

CLASS 3: ASSESS RISK & TAKE ACTION IF NECESSARY
- *Consider Alternative*: Use an alternative to the enzyme inhibitor if possible.
  Calcium channel blockers: Calcium channel blockers other than diltiazem and verapamil are unlikely to inhibit CYP3A4.
  Grapefruit: Orange juice does not appear to inhibit CYP3A4.
- *Circumvent/Minimize*: Consider reducing the dose of the protease inhibitor if enzyme inhibitors are coadministered.
- *Monitor*: Monitor for protease inhibitor toxicity.

OBJECT DRUGS	PRECIPITANT DRUGS	
Quetiapine	**Enzyme Inducers:**	
(Seroquel)	**Barbiturates**	**Phenytoin** (Dilantin)
	Bosentan (Tracleer)	**Primidone** (Mysoline)
	Carbamazepine	**Rifabutin** (Mycobutin)
	(Tegretol)	**Rifampin** (Rifadin)
	Efavirenz (Sustiva)	**Rifapentine** (Priftin)
	Nevirapine (Viramune)	**St. John's Wort**
	Oxcarbazepine (Trileptal)	

COMMENTS: Enzyme inducers may reduce the serum levels of quetiapine resulting in loss of efficacy. The effect can be large; for example, carbamazepine has been shown to dramatically reduce quetiapine concentrations, sometimes to undetectable levels.

CLASS 2: USE ONLY IF BENEFIT FELT TO OUTWEIGH RISK
- *Use Alternative*:
  Enzyme Inducer: Use an alternative to the enzyme inducer if possible.
  Quetiapine: Most other atypical antipsychotics are metabolized by CYP3A4 or CYP1A2, and are likely to be similarly affected by enzyme inducers.
- *Circumvent/Minimize*: Consider increasing the dose of the quetiapine if enzyme inducers are coadministered. Unfortunately, due to the potentially large magnitude of the interaction, it may not be practical to increase the quetiapine dose enough to achieve an adequate response. If the quetiapine dose is increased to compensate for the enzyme induction, discontinuation of the enzyme inducer with continued quetiapine therapy is likely to result in excessive quetiapine concentrations.
- *Monitor*: If it is necessary to use quetiapine with enzyme inducers, monitor for loss of quetiapine efficacy; measuring quetiapine plasma concentrations may be necessary. Keep in mind that enzyme induction is usually gradual and may take days to weeks for onset and offset, depending on the specific inducer.

OBJECT DRUGS	PRECIPITANT DRUGS	
Quetiapine	**Antimicrobials:**	
(Seroquel)	**Clarithromycin** (Biaxin)	**Posaconazole** (Noxafil)
	Erythromycin (E-Mycin)	**Quinupristin** (Synercid)
	Fluconazole (Diflucan)	**Telithromycin** (Ketek)
	Itraconazole (Sporanox)	**Troleandomycin** (TAO)
	Ketoconazole (Nizoral)	**Voriconazole** (Vfend)

COMMENTS: Quetiapine is metabolized primarily by CYP3A4, and inhibitors of CYP3A4 may increase the serum levels of quetiapine. For example, in one study the potent CYP3A4 inhibitor ketoconazole produced more than a 5-fold increase in quetiapine plasma concentrations. Clarithromycin, another potent CYP3A4 inhibitor, has produced severe quetiapine toxicity.

CLASS 3: ASSESS RISK & TAKE ACTION IF NECESSARY
- *Consider Alternative*:
  Azole Antifungals: Itraconazole and ketoconazole are potent inhibitors of CYP3A4; fluconazole appears weaker, but in larger doses it also inhibits CYP3A4. **Terbinafine** (Lamisil) does not appear to affect CYP3A4, and would not be expected to interact with quetiapine. (Terbinafine inhibits CYP2D6, but quetiapine metabolism by CYP2D6 appears to be minimal.)
  Macrolide Antibiotics: Unlike erythromycin, clarithromycin and troleandomycin, **azithromycin** (Zithromax) and **dirithromycin*** do not appear to inhibit CYP3A4. (*not available in US)
  Telithromycin: The use of **azithromycin** (Zithromax) or a quinolone antibiotic may be considered.
- *Circumvent/Minimize*: Consider reducing the dose of quetiapine if enzyme inhibitors are coadministered.
- *Monitor*: Monitor for quetiapine toxicity such as excessive sedation, confusion, hypotension, respiratory depression, dizziness, and fainting.

OBJECT DRUGS	PRECIPITANT DRUGS
Quetiapine (Seroquel)	**Antidepressants:** **Fluvoxamine** (Luvox) **Nefazodone**

COMMENTS: Quetiapine is metabolized primarily by CYP3A4, and drugs that inhibit CYP3A4 may increase the serum levels of quetiapine. Nefazodone is also a potent inhibitor of CYP3A4, and may also produce large increases. Fluvoxamine is generally less potent as a CYP3A4 inhibitor, and it has been associated with moderate increases in quetiapine plasma concentrations.

CLASS 3: ASSESS RISK & TAKE ACTION IF NECESSARY
- *Consider Alternative*: **Sertraline** (Zoloft), **citalopram** (Celexa), **escitalopram** (Lexapro), **venlafaxine** (Effexor), and **paroxetine** (Paxil) appear less likely to inhibit CYP3A4 than fluvoxamine. **Fluoxetine** (Prozac) appears to be a weak inhibitor of CYP3A4, but available clinical evidence suggests that fluoxetine (as well as most other SSRIs) have little or no effect on plasma quetiapine concentrations.
- *Circumvent/Minimize*: Consider reducing the dose of quetiapine if enzyme inhibitors are coadministered.
- *Monitor*: Monitor for quetiapine toxicity such as excessive sedation, confusion, hypotension, respiratory depression, dizziness, and fainting.

OBJECT DRUGS	PRECIPITANT DRUGS	
Quetiapine (Seroquel)	**Enzyme Inhibitors:**	
	Amiodarone (Cordarone)	**Diltiazem** (Cardizem)
	Amprenavir (Agenerase)	**Grapefruit**
	Aprepitant (Emend)	**Indinavir** (Crixivan)
	Atazanavir (Reyataz)	**Nelfinavir** (Viracept)
	Conivaptan (Vaprisol)	**Ritonavir** (Norvir)
	Cyclosporine (Neoral)	**Saquinavir** (Invirase)
	Darunavir (Prezista)	**Verapamil** (Isoptin)
	Delavirdine (Rescriptor)	

COMMENTS: Quetiapine is metabolized primarily by CYP3A4, and drugs that inhibit CYP3A4 may increase the serum levels of quetiapine.

CLASS 3: ASSESS RISK & TAKE ACTION IF NECESSARY
- *Consider Alternative*: Use an alternative to the enzyme inhibitor if possible.
  Calcium channel blockers: Calcium channel blockers other than diltiazem and verapamil are unlikely to inhibit CYP3A4.
  Grapefruit: Orange juice does not appear to inhibit CYP3A4.
- *Circumvent/Minimize*: Consider reducing the dose of the quetiapine if enzyme inhibitors are coadministered.
- *Monitor*: Monitor for quetiapine toxicity such as excessive sedation, confusion, hypotension, respiratory depression, dizziness, and fainting.

OBJECT DRUGS	PRECIPITANT DRUGS
Quinolones:	**Binding Agents:**
Ciprofloxacin (Cipro)	**Antacids**
Enoxacin (Penetrex)	**Calcium Polycarbophil** (FiberCon)
Gemifloxacin (Factive)	**Didanosine** (Videx)
Levofloxacin (Levaquin)	**Iron**
Lomefloxacin (Maxaquin)	**Sucralfate** (Carafate)
Moxifloxacin (Avelox)	**Zinc**
Norfloxacin (Noroxin)	
Ofloxacin (Floxin)	
Sparfloxacin (Zagam)	

COMMENTS: The absorption of quinolones is markedly reduced by agents containing cations such as aluminum, magnesium, and to a lesser extent, iron and calcium. Ciprofloxacin and norfloxacin appear more susceptible to this effect than lomefloxacin or ofloxacin; iron has little effect on lomefloxacin and ofloxacin. Limited evidence suggests that the absorption of some quinolones may be affected by multivitamins with minerals.

CLASS 3: ASSESS RISK & TAKE ACTION IF NECESSARY

- *Consider Alternative*: Calcium carbonate does not impair quinolone absorption as much as aluminum-magnesium antacids, but it would still be prudent to separate doses. Gatifloxacin absorption does not appear to be affected by calcium carbonate. Enteric coated didanosine (Videx EC) does not interact.
- *Circumvent/Minimize*: Giving the quinolone 2 hours before or 6 hours after the cation minimizes the interaction.
- *Monitor*: Watch for reduced quinolone antibiotic efficacy in patients taking di- or trivalent cations.

OBJECT DRUGS	PRECIPITANT DRUGS	
Ranolazine (Ranexa)	**Antimicrobials:**	
	Clarithromycin (Biaxin)	**Posaconazole** (Noxafil)
	Erythromycin (E-Mycin)	**Quinupristin** (Synercid)
	Fluconazole (Diflucan)	**Telithromycin** (Ketek)
	Itraconazole (Sporanox)	**Troleandomycin** (TAO)
	Ketoconazole (Nizoral)	**Voriconazole** (Vfend)

COMMENTS: Ranolazine is metabolized primarily by CYP3A4, and inhibitors of this isozyme increase the serum concentrations of ranolazine. The product information states that ranolazine is contraindicated with potent or moderately potent CYP3A4 inhibitors. Theoretically, such drugs could increase the risk of ranolazine-induced QTc prolongation and ventricular arrhythmias.

CLASS 2: USE ONLY IF BENEFIT FELT TO OUTWEIGH RISK

- *Use Alternative*:
  Azole Antifungals: Itraconazole and ketoconazole are potent inhibitors of CYP3A4; fluconazole appears weaker, but in larger doses it also inhibits CYP3A4.

<u>Macrolide Antibiotics</u>: Unlike erythromycin, clarithromycin and troleandomycin, **azithromycin** (Zithromax) and **dirithromycin*** do not appear to inhibit CYP3A4. (*not available in US)

<u>Telithromycin</u>: The use of **azithromycin** (Zithromax) or a quinolone antibiotic may be considered.

- ***Circumvent/Minimize***: Consider reducing the dose of ranolazine if enzyme inhibitors are coadministered.
- ***Monitor***: If the combination is used, the primary concern is QTc prolongation. Monitor the ECG and advise the patient to report any episodes of dizziness or syncope.

OBJECT DRUGS	PRECIPITANT DRUGS
Ranolazine (Ranexa)	<u>**Antidepressants:**</u> **Fluvoxamine** (Luvox) **Nefazodone**

COMMENTS: Ranolazine is metabolized primarily by CYP3A4, and inhibitors of this isozyme increase the serum concentrations of ranolazine. The product information states that ranolazine is contraindicated with potent (nefazodone) or moderately potent (fluvoxamine) CYP3A4 inhibitors. Theoretically, such drugs could increase the risk of ranolazine-induced QTc prolongation and ventricular arrhythmias.

CLASS 2: USE ONLY IF BENEFIT FELT TO OUTWEIGH RISK

- ***Consider Alternative***: **Sertraline** (Zoloft), **citalopram** (Celexa), **escitalopram** (Lexapro), and **venlafaxine** (Effexor), have little effect on CYP3A4.
- ***Circumvent/Minimize***: Consider reducing the dose of ranolazine if enzyme inhibitors are coadministered.
- ***Monitor***: If the combination is used, the primary concern is QTc prolongation. Monitor the ECG and advise the patient to report any episodes of dizziness or syncope.

OBJECT DRUGS	PRECIPITANT DRUGS	
Ranolazine (Ranexa)	<u>**Enzyme Inhibitors:**</u>	
	Amiodarone (Cordarone)	**Diltiazem** (Cardizem)
	Amprenavir (Agenerase)	**Grapefruit**
	Aprepitant (Emend)	**Indinavir** (Crixivan)
	Atazanavir (Reyataz)	**Nelfinavir** (Viracept)
	Conivaptan (Vaprisol)	**Ritonavir** (Norvir)
	Cyclosporine (Neoral)	**Saquinavir** (Invirase)
	Darunavir (Prezista)	**Verapamil** (Isoptin)
	Delavirdine (Rescriptor)	

COMMENTS: Ranolazine is metabolized primarily by CYP3A4, and inhibitors of this isozyme increase the serum concentrations of ranolazine. The product information states that ranolazine is contraindicated with potent or moderately potent CYP3A4 inhibitors. Theoretically, such drugs could increase the risk of ranolazine-induced QTc prolongation and ventricular arrhythmias. Because

amiodarone inhibits CYP3A4 and also intrinsically prolongs the QTc interval, it would be wise to avoid combining it with ranolazine (**Class 1**).

CLASS 2: USE ONLY IF BENEFIT FELT TO OUTWEIGH RISK
- *Use Alternative*: Use an alternative to the enzyme inhibitor if possible.
  Calcium channel blockers: Calcium channel blockers other than diltiazem and verapamil are unlikely to inhibit CYP3A4.
  Grapefruit: Orange juice does not appear to inhibit CYP3A4.
- *Circumvent/Minimize*: Consider reducing the dose of the ranolazine if enzyme inhibitors are coadministered.
- *Monitor:* If the combination is used, the primary concern is QTc prolongation. Monitor the ECG and advise the patient to report any episodes of dizziness or syncope.

OBJECT DRUGS	PRECIPITANT DRUGS
Rifabutin (Mycobutin)	**Antidepressants:**
	Fluvoxamine (Luvox)
	Nefazodone

COMMENTS: Rifabutin serum concentrations can be markedly increased by CYP3A4 inhibitors; toxicity is often manifested by uveitis but rash, bone marrow suppression, and increased hepatic enzymes can also occur.

CLASS 2: USE ONLY IF BENEFIT FELT TO OUTWEIGH RISK
- *Consider Alternative*: **Sertraline** (Zoloft), **citalopram** (Celexa), **escitalopram** (Lexapro), **venlafaxine** (Effexor), and **paroxetine** (Paxil) appear less likely to inhibit CYP3A4. **Fluoxetine** (Prozac) appears to be a weak inhibitor of CYP3A4.
- *Circumvent/Minimize*: Rifabutin dose may require reduction if used with CYP3A4 inhibitors.
- *Monitor:* If CYP3A4 inhibitors are used with rifabutin, monitor for rifabutin toxicity.

OBJECT DRUGS	PRECIPITANT DRUGS	
Rifabutin	**Antimicrobials:**	
(Mycobutin)	**Clarithromycin** (Biaxin)	**Posaconazole** (Noxafil)
	Erythromycin (E-Mycin)	**Quinupristin** (Synercid)
	Fluconazole (Diflucan)	**Telithromycin** (Ketek)
	Itraconazole (Sporanox)	**Troleandomycin** (TAO)
	Ketoconazole (Nizoral)	**Voriconazole** (Vfend)

COMMENTS: Rifabutin serum concentrations can be markedly increased by CYP3A4 inhibitors; toxicity is often manifested by uveitis but rash, bone marrow suppression, and increased hepatic enzymes can also occur. Also, rifabutin may substantially reduce plasma concentrations of clarithromycin, and probably also most of the other antimicrobials listed.

CLASS 2: USE ONLY IF BENEFIT FELT TO OUTWEIGH RISK
- *Use Alternative*:
  Azole Antifungals: Itraconazole and ketoconazole are potent inhibitors of CYP3A4; fluconazole appears weaker, but in larger doses it also inhibits

CYP3A4. **Terbinafine** (Lamisil) does not appear to affect CYP3A4, and would not be expected to interact with rifabutin.

Macrolide Antibiotics: Unlike erythromycin, clarithromycin and troleandomycin, **azithromycin** (Zithromax) and **dirithromycin*** do not appear to inhibit CYP3A4. (*not available in US)

Telithromycin: The use of **azithromycin** (Zithromax) or a quinolone antibiotic should be considered.

- ***Circumvent/Minimize***: Rifabutin dose may require reduction if used with CYP3A4 inhibitors.
- ***Monitor***: If CYP3A4 inhibitors are used with rifabutin, monitor for rifabutin toxicity, especially uveitis.

OBJECT DRUGS	PRECIPITANT DRUGS	
Rifabutin	**Enzyme Inhibitors:**	
(Mycobutin)	**Amiodarone** (Cordarone)	**Diltiazem** (Cardizem)
	Amprenavir (Agenerase)	**Grapefruit**
	Aprepitant (Emend)	**Indinavir** (Crixivan)
	Atazanavir (Reyataz)	**Nelfinavir** (Viracept)
	Conivaptan (Vaprisol)	**Ritonavir** (Norvir)
	Cyclosporine (Neoral)	**Saquinavir** (Invirase)
	Darunavir (Prezista)	**Verapamil** (Isoptin)
	Delavirdine (Rescriptor)	

COMMENTS: Rifabutin serum concentrations can be markedly increased by CYP3A4 inhibitors; toxicity is often manifested by uveitis but rash, bone marrow suppression, and increased hepatic enzymes can also occur. Also, the plasma concentrations of some of the enzyme inhibitors listed above (e.g., cyclosporine, diltiazem, verapamil) are likely to be substantially reduced due to the ability of rifabutin to act as an enzyme inducer.

CLASS 2: USE ONLY IF BENEFIT FELT TO OUTWEIGH RISK

- ***Use Alternative***:
  Enzyme Inhibitor: Use an alternative to the enzyme inhibitor if possible.
  Calcium Channel Blockers: Calcium channel blockers other than diltiazem and verapamil are unlikely to inhibit the metabolism of rifabutin. But most calcium channel blockers are highly susceptible to enzyme induction, so rifabutin is likely to substantially reduce their plasma concentrations.
  Grapefruit: Orange juice does not appear to inhibit CYP3A4.
- ***Circumvent/Minimize***: Rifabutin dose may require reduction if used with CYP3A4 inhibitors. In patients on ritonavir, the use of rifabutin once or twice weekly has been successful in some patients.
- ***Monitor***: If CYP3A4 inhibitors are used with rifabutin, monitor for rifabutin toxicity.

OBJECT DRUGS	PRECIPITANT DRUGS
Sildenafil (Viagra)	**Antidepressants:**
Tadalafil (Cialis)	**Fluvoxamine** (Luvox)
Vardenafil (Levitra)	**Nefazodone**

COMMENTS: The phosphodiesterase inhibitors are metabolized by CYP3A4 and concurrent administration with CYP3A4 inhibitors could produce increased plasma concentrations. Increased side effects may occur during coadministered with CYP3A4 inhibitors.

CLASS 3: ASSESS RISK & TAKE ACTION IF NECESSARY
- *Consider Alternative*: Sertraline (Zoloft), **venlafaxine** (Effexor), **paroxetine** (Paxil), **citalopram** (Celexa), and **escitalopram** (Lexapro) are not known to inhibit CYP3A4. **Fluoxetine** (Prozac) appears to be a weak inhibitor of CYP3A4.
- *Monitor*: Monitor for phosphodiesterase inhibitor toxicity including visual disturbances, hypotension, and syncope. Reduced dose of the phosphodiesterase inhibitor may be required.

OBJECT DRUGS	PRECIPITANT DRUGS	
Sildenafil (Viagra)	<u>Antimicrobials:</u>	
Tadalafil (Cialis)	**Clarithromycin** (Biaxin)	**Posaconazole** (Noxafil)
Vardenafil (Levitra)	**Erythromycin** (E-Mycin)	**Quinupristin** (Synercid)
	Fluconazole (Diflucan)	**Telithromycin** (Ketek)
	Itraconazole (Sporanox)	**Troleandomycin** (TAO)
	Ketoconazole (Nizoral)	**Voriconazole** (Vfend)

COMMENTS: The phosphodiesterase inhibitors appear to be metabolized by CYP3A4 and concurrent administration with CYP3A4 inhibitors could produce increased plasma concentrations. Increased side effects may occur during coadministered with CYP3A4 inhibitors.

CLASS 3: ASSESS RISK & TAKE ACTION IF NECESSARY
- *Consider Alternative*:
  Azole Antifungals: Itraconazole and ketoconazole are potent inhibitors of CYP3A4; fluconazole appears weaker, but in larger doses it also inhibits CYP3A4. **Terbinafine** (Lamisil) does not appear to affect CYP3A4, and would not be expected to interact with phosphodiesterase inhibitors.
  Macrolide Antibiotics: Unlike erythromycin, clarithromycin and troleandomycin, **azithromycin** (Zithromax) and **dirithromycin*** do not appear to inhibit CYP3A4. (*not available in US)
  Telithromycin: The use of **azithromycin** (Zithromax) or a quinolone antibiotic should be considered.
- *Monitor*: Monitor for phosphodiesterase inhibitor toxicity including visual disturbances, hypotension, and syncope. Reduced dose of the phosphodiesterase inhibitor may be required.

OBJECT DRUGS	PRECIPITANT DRUGS
Sildenafil (Viagra)	<u>Calcium Channel Blockers:</u>
Tadalafil (Cialis)	**Diltiazem** (Cardizem)
Vardenafil (Levitra)	**Verapamil** (Isoptin)

COMMENTS: The phosphodiesterase inhibitors appear to be metabolized by CYP3A4 and concurrent administration with CYP3A4 inhibitors such as diltiazem and verapamil could produce increased plasma concentrations. Increased side effects may occur during coadministered with CYP3A4 inhibitors.

CLASS 3: ASSESS RISK & TAKE ACTION IF NECESSARY
- ***Consider Alternative***: Calcium channel blockers other than diltiazem and verapamil are unlikely to inhibit the metabolism of sildenafil. However, other calcium channel blockers may produce increased hypotensive effects when used with phosphodiesterase inhibitors.
- ***Monitor***: Monitor for phosphodiesterase inhibitor toxicity including visual disturbances, hypotension, and syncope. Reduced dose of the phosphodiesterase inhibitor may be required.

OBJECT DRUGS	PRECIPITANT DRUGS	
Sildenafil (Viagra)	**Enzyme Inhibitors:**	
Tadalafil (Cialis)	**Amiodarone** (Cordarone)	**Darunavir** (Prezista)
Vardenafil (Levitra)	**Amprenavir** (Agenerase)	**Delavirdine** (Rescriptor)
	Aprepitant (Emend)	**Grapefruit**
	Atazanavir (Reyataz)	**Indinavir** (Crixivan)
	Cimetidine (Tagamet)	**Nelfinavir** (Viracept)
	Conivaptan (Vaprisol)	**Ritonavir** (Norvir)
	Cyclosporine (Neoral)	**Saquinavir** (Invirase)

COMMENTS: The phosphodiesterase inhibitors appear to be metabolized by CYP3A4 and concurrent administration with CYP3A4 inhibitors could produce increased plasma concentrations. Increased side effects may occur during coadministration with CYP3A4 inhibitors.

CLASS 3: ASSESS RISK & TAKE ACTION IF NECESSARY
- ***Consider Alternative***:
  Cimetidine: **Famotidine** (Pepcid), **nizatidine** (Axid), and **ranitidine** (Zantac) have minimal effects on drug metabolism.
  Grapefruit: Orange juice does not appear to inhibit CYP3A4.
- ***Monitor***: Monitor for phosphodiesterase inhibitor toxicity including visual disturbances, hypotension, and syncope. Reduced dose of the phosphodiesterase inhibitor may be required.

OBJECT DRUGS	PRECIPITANT DRUGS
Tamoxifen (Nolvadex)	**Antidepressants**:
	Bupropion (Wellbutrin)
	Duloxetine (Cymbalta)
	Fluoxetine (Prozac)
	Paroxetine (Paxil)

COMMENTS: Tamoxifen is a prodrug that is converted to active metabolites by CYP2D6. Evidence from studies in patients with breast cancer have shown that patients on potent CYP2D6 inhibitors have reduced concentrations of active tamoxifen metabolites, and reduced survival. People with "normal" CYP2D6 activity ("Rapid Metabolizers") will be at the greatest risk.

CLASS 2: USE ONLY IF BENEFIT FELT TO OUTWEIGH RISK

- *Use Alternative*:

  <u>Antidepressant</u>: Given the severity of the potential interaction, every effort should be made to avoid the above antidepressants in patients receiving tamoxifen. Alternative antidepressants have less effect on CYP2D6: **citalopram** (Celexa), **desvenlafaxine** (Pristiq), **escitalopram** (Lexapro), and **sertraline** (Zoloft), are weak inhibitors of CYP2D6, and **fluvoxamine** and **venlafaxine** (Effexor) have little or no effect on CYP2D6.

- *Monitor*: If CYP2D6 inhibitors are used with tamoxifen, be alert for evidence of reduced tamoxifen effect.

OBJECT DRUGS	PRECIPITANT DRUGS	
Tamoxifen	**Enzyme Inhibitors:**	
(Nolvadex)	**Amiodarone** (Cordarone)	**Propoxyphene** (Darvon)
	Cimetidine (Tagamet)	**Quinidine** (Quinidex)
	Cinacalcet (Sensipar)	**Ritonavir** (Norvir)
	Diphenhydramine (Benadryl)	**Terbinafine** (Lamisil)
	Haloperidol (Haldol)	**Thioridazine** (Mellaril)
	Propafenone (Rythmol)	

COMMENTS: Tamoxifen is a prodrug that is converted to active metabolites by CYP2D6. Studies in patients with breast cancer have shown that patients on potent CYP2D6 inhibitors have reduced concentrations of active tamoxifen metabolites, and reduced survival. People with "normal" CYP2D6 activity ("Rapid Metabolizers") will be at the greatest risk from these interactions. Note that because terbinafine has an extraordinarily long terminal half-life, the inhibitory effect of terbinafine on CYP2D6 may last for many weeks after terbinafine is discontinued.

CLASS 2: USE ONLY IF BENEFIT FELT TO OUTWEIGH RISK

- *Use Alternative*:

  <u>Cimetidine</u>: **Famotidine** (Pepcid), **nizatidine** (Axid), and **ranitidine** (Zantac) have minimal effects on drug metabolism.

  <u>Diphenhydramine</u>: Other antihistamines such as **desloratadine** (Clarinex), **fexofenadine** (Allegra), **loratadine** Claritin), and **cetirizine** (Zyrtec) are not known to inhibit CYP2D6.

  <u>Propoxyphene</u>: Consider using an alternative analgesic; propoxyphene has limited efficacy, and other analgesics appear less likely to affect CYP2D6.

- *Monitor*: If CYP2D6 inhibitors are used with tamoxifen, be alert for evidence of reduced tamoxifen effect.

OBJECT DRUGS	PRECIPITANT DRUGS
Tetracyclines:	**Absorption Inhibitors:**
Demeclocycline (Declomycin)	**Antacids**
Doxycycline (Vibramycin)	**Bismuth** (Pepto Bismol)
Minocycline (Minocin)	**Didanosine** (Videx)
Oxytetracycline	**Iron**
Tetracycline	**Sucralfate** (Carafate)
	Zinc

COMMENTS: The absorption of tetracyclines may be reduced by agents containing cations such as aluminum, magnesium, and to a lesser extent, iron. Doxycycline may be less susceptible to these interactions than other tetracyclines, and does not appear to be affected significantly by iron.

CLASS 3: ASSESS RISK & TAKE ACTION IF NECESSARY

- *Circumvent/Minimize*: Give the tetracycline 2 hours before or 6 hours after the absorption inhibitor to minimize the interaction. Enteric coated didanosine (Videx EC) does not appear to interact.
- *Monitor*: Watch for reduced tetracycline efficacy in patients taking absorption inhibitors.

OBJECT DRUGS	PRECIPITANT DRUGS	
Theophylline	**Enzyme Inducers:**	
	Barbiturates	**Phenytoin** (Dilantin)
	Bosentan (Tracleer)	**Primidone** (Mysoline)
	Carbamazepine (Tegretol)	**Rifabutin** (Mycobutin)
	Efavirenz (Sustiva)	**Rifampin** (Rifadin)
	Griseofulvin	**Rifapentine** (Priftin)
	Nevirapine (Viramune)	**St. John's Wort**
	Oxcarbazepine (Trileptal)	

COMMENTS: Enzyme inducers enhance the metabolism of theophylline by CYP3A4 and probably also CYP1A2, thus reducing theophylline serum concentrations. Higher than usual theophylline doses may be needed in the presence of an enzyme inducer. Accordingly, serious theophylline toxicity has been reported following discontinuation of an enzyme inducer in patients stabilized on theophylline.

CLASS 3: ASSESS RISK & TAKE ACTION IF NECESSARY

- *Monitor*: Monitor for altered theophylline serum concentrations if an enzyme inducer is initiated, discontinued, or changed in dosage.

OBJECT DRUGS	PRECIPITANT DRUGS
Theophylline	Fluvoxamine (Luvox)

COMMENTS: Theophylline is metabolized by CYP1A2 and to a lesser extent CYP3A4. Fluvoxamine is a potent inhibitor of CYP1A2, and may produce dramatic increases in theophylline plasma concentrations; theophylline toxicity is likely to occur.

CLASS 2: USE ONLY IF BENEFIT FELT TO OUTWEIGH RISK

- *Use Alternative*: Sertraline (Zoloft), **fluoxetine** (Prozac), **venlafaxine** (Effexor), **paroxetine** (Paxil), **citalopram** (Celexa), and **escitalopram** (Lexapro) are not known to inhibit CYP1A2. **Nefazodone** is a potent inhibitor of CYP3A4, and may increase theophylline concentrations, but probably to a lesser extent than fluvoxamine.
- *Monitor*: Monitor for altered theophylline response if a CYP1A2 inhibitor is initiated, discontinued, or the dose is changed. Evidence of theophylline toxicity includes nausea, vomiting, diarrhea, restlessness, irritability, and

insomnia. Higher serum concentrations can result in cardiac arrhythmias or seizures.

OBJECT DRUGS	PRECIPITANT DRUGS
Theophylline	**Antimicrobials:**
	Ciprofloxacin (Cipro)
	Clarithromycin (Biaxin)
	Enoxacin (Penetrex)
	Erythromycin (E-Mycin)
	Troleandomycin (TAO)

COMMENTS: Theophylline is metabolized by CYP1A2 and to a lesser extent CYP3A4. Inhibitors of these isozymes can increase theophylline serum concentrations; some patients may develop theophylline toxicity. Ciprofloxacin and especially enoxacin are strong inhibitors of CYP1A2, and can produce serious theophylline toxicity. Clarithromycin, erythromycin, and troleandomycin usually do not increase theophylline concentrations as much, but toxicity can still occur.

CLASS 2: USE ONLY IF BENEFIT FELT TO OUTWEIGH RISK

- *Use Alternative*:
  Macrolides: Unlike erythromycin, clarithromycin and troleandomycin, **azithromycin** (Zithromax) and **dirithromycin*** do not inhibit CYP450 isozymes. (*not available in US)
  Quinolones: **Levofloxacin** (Levaquin), **lomefloxacin** (Maxaquin), **ofloxacin** (Floxin), and **moxifloxacin** (Avelox) appear to have little effect on CYP1A2 or CYP3A4.
- *Monitor*: Monitor for altered theophylline response if a CYP1A2 inhibitor is initiated, discontinue, or the dose is changed. Evidence of theophylline toxicity includes nausea, vomiting, diarrhea, restlessness, irritability, and insomnia. Higher serum concentrations can result in cardiac arrhythmias or seizures.

OBJECT DRUGS	PRECIPITANT DRUGS	
Theophylline	**Enzyme Inhibitors:**	
	Allopurinol (Zyloprim)	**Mexiletine** (Mexitil)
	(600mg/day or more)	**Pentoxifylline** (Trental)
	Atazanavir (Reyataz)	**Tacrine** (Cognex)
	Cimetidine (Tagamet)	**Thiabendazole** (Mintezol)
	Disulfiram (Antabuse)	**Ticlopidine** (Ticlid)
	Febuxostat (Uloric)	**Zileuton** (Zyflo)

COMMENTS: Inhibitors of CYP1A2 (and to a lesser extent CYP3A4) may increase serum theophylline concentrations; some patients may develop theophylline toxicity. These inhibitors appear to have less risk of serious theophylline toxicity than the interaction on the previous pages, and/or these are no obvious alternatives to use in their place. Febuxostat is a xanthine oxidase inhibitor, and theophylline is partially metabolized by xanthine oxidase. Although this interaction is based primarily on theoretical considerations, the manufacturer states that the combination is contraindicated.

- *Consider Alternative*: Use an alternative to the enzyme inhibitor if possible.
  Cimetidine: Although the cimetidine-theophylline interaction is usually modest, an alternative is preferable. **Famotidine** (Pepcid), **nizatidine** (Axid), and **ranitidine** (Zantac) have minimal effects on drug metabolism.
- *Monitor*: Monitor for altered theophylline response if a CYP1A2 inhibitor is initiated, discontinued, or the dose is changed. Evidence of theophylline toxicity includes nausea, vomiting, diarrhea, restlessness, irritability, and insomnia. Higher serum concentrations can result in cardiac arrhythmias or seizures.

OBJECT DRUGS	PRECIPITANT DRUGS	
Thiazide Diuretics	**SSRI and SNRI:**	
	Citalopram (Celexa)	**Fluvoxamine** (Luvox)
	Clomipramine (Anafranil)	**Imipramine** (Tofranil)
	Desvenlafaxine (Pristiq)	**Milnacipran** (Savella)
	Duloxetine (Cymbalta)	**Paroxetine** (Paxil)
	Escitalopram (Lexapro)	**Sertraline** (Zoloft)
	Fluoxetine (Prozac)	**Venlafaxine** (Effexor)

COMMENTS: Selective serotonin reuptake inhibitors (SSRI) and selective serotonin/norepinephrine reuptake inhibitors (SNRI) have been reported to cause syndrome of inappropriate antidiuretic hormone (SIADH) with hyponatremia. Thiazide diuretics increase sodium excretion, and can have additive hyponatremic effects.

CLASS 3: ASSESS RISK & TAKE ACTION IF NECESSARY

- *Consider Alternative*:
  Antidepressants: Some evidence suggests that **mirtazapine** (Remeron) is less likely to cause hyponatremia, but more evidence is needed.
- *Monitor*: Monitor for symptoms of hyponatremia: confusion, disorientation, nausea, headache, weakness, fatigue, muscle cramps. If the hyponatremia is severe, it can lead to seizures, coma and death. In predisposed patients such as elderly women it may be prudent to measure baseline serum sodium and again a week or so after the second drug was started. Hyponatremia usually occurs within 2 to 3 weeks of starting therapy of adding the second drug.

OBJECT DRUGS	PRECIPITANT DRUGS
Thioridazine (Mellaril)	**Drugs That Inhibit CYP2D6 and Prolong the QT Interval:**
	Amiodarone (Cordarone)
	Dronedarone (Multaq)
	Haloperidol (Haldol)
	Propafenone (Rythmol)
	Quinidine (Quinidex)
	Ranolazine (Ranexa)

COMMENTS: Thioridazine can prolong the QT interval in a dose-dependent manner. Drugs that inhibit the cytochrome P450 isozymes involved in thioridazine metabolism (primarily CYP2D6) may increase the risk of ventricular arrhythmias such as torsades de pointes. Amiodarone and quinidine are strong inhibitors of CYP2D6, and also individually prolong the QT interval. Hence, the risk of serious arrhythmias is likely to be substantially increased. The product information for thioridazine states that it is contraindicated with known CYP2D6 inhibitors or drugs that increase the QT interval.

CLASS 1: AVOID COMBINATION

- *Avoid*: Avoid the use of amiodarone or quinidine in patients receiving thioridazine.
- *Use Alternative*:
  Thioridazine: Most other phenothiazines produce less QT prolongation than thioridazine. **Pimozide** (Orap) can substantially prolong the QT interval and would not be a suitable substitute for thioridazine.
  Antiarrhythmics: It may be difficult to find an alternative antiarrhythmic that can be used safely with thioridazine. Several other antiarrhythmics such as **disopyramide** (Norpace), **procainamide** (Pronestyl), and **sotalol** (Betapace) can prolong the QT interval, and should be used only with extreme caution with thioridazine.
- *Monitor*: If combined therapy is necessary, monitor carefully for signs of delayed ventricular repolarization (prolonged QT interval) and symptoms of torsades de pointes including palpitations and syncope.

OBJECT DRUGS	PRECIPITANT DRUGS	
Thioridazine (Mellaril)	**Enzyme Inhibitors:**	
	Bupropion (Wellbutrin)	**Fluvoxamine** (Luvox)
	Chloroquine	**Haloperidol** (Haldol)
	Cimetidine (Tagamet)	**Paroxetine** (Paxil)
	Cinacalcet (Sensipar)	**Propoxyphene** (Darvon)
	Diphenhydramine (Benadryl)	**Ritonavir** (Norvir)
	Duloxetine (Cymbalta)	**Terbinafine** (Lamisil)
	Fluoxetine (Prozac)	

COMMENTS: Thioridazine can prolong the QT interval. Inhibitors of CYP2D6 may increase the risk of ventricular arrhythmias such as torsades de pointes. The product information for thioridazine states that concurrent use with known CYP2D6 inhibitors (or fluvoxamine) is contraindicated. Note that because terbinafine has an extraordinarily long terminal half-life, the inhibitory effect of terbinafine on CYP2D6 may last for many weeks after terbinafine is discontinued.

CLASS 2: USE ONLY IF BENEFIT FELT TO OUTWEIGH RISK

- *Use Alternative*: Use an alternative to the enzyme inhibitor if possible.
  Antidepressants: **Citalopram** (Celexa), **escitalopram** (Lexapro), **sertraline** (Zoloft), and **desvenlafaxine** (Pristiq), **venlafaxine** (Effexor) have less effect on CYP2D6 than fluoxetine and paroxetine, and would not be expected to have a large effect on thioridazine metabolism.

<u>Cimetidine</u>: **Famotidine** (Pepcid), **nizatidine** (Axid), and **ranitidine** (Zantac) have no known effects on CYP2D6 activity.

<u>Thioridazine</u>: Most other phenothiazines produce less QT prolongation than thioridazine. **Pimozide** (Orap) can substantially prolong the QT interval and would not be a suitable substitute for thioridazine.

- *Monitor*: If combined therapy is necessary, monitor carefully for signs of delayed ventricular repolarization (prolonged QT interval) and symptoms of torsades de pointes including palpitations and syncope.

OBJECT DRUGS	PRECIPITANT DRUGS
Thyroid:	**Binding Agents:**
Levothyroxine (Synthroid)	**Antacids**
Liothyronine (Cytomel)	**Cholestyramine** (Questran)
Liotrix (Thyrolar)	**Colestipol** (Colestid)
Thyroid USP	**Iron**
	Sevelamer (Renagel)
	Sucralfate (Carafate)

COMMENTS: Antacids (calcium, aluminum, magnesium), cholestyramine, colestipol, sevelamer, and possibly iron can inhibit thyroid hormone absorption if given concurrently. There is a large variability in the magnitude of this interaction from one person to another, probably because some people on thyroid have some residual thyroid function. The effect of **colesevelam** (Welchol) and **ezetimibe** (Zetia) on thyroid hormone absorption is not established, but some evidence suggests that these agents are less likely to bind with other drugs than cholestyramine and colestipol. Limited evidence suggests that thyroxine absorption may also be inhibited by **ciprofloxacin (Cipro)**, **caffeine**, and **sertraline** (Zoloft), but more evidence is needed to assess the clinical importance of these interactions.

CLASS 3: **ASSESS RISK & TAKE ACTION IF NECESSARY**

- *Circumvent/Minimize*: Minimize interactions by giving thyroid 2 hours before or 6 hours after the binding agent; keep a constant interval between doses of thyroid and binding agents. Some reduction in thyroid levels may still occur due to enterohepatic circulation of thyroxine.
- *Monitor*: Monitor If thyroid hormones are administered with binding agents, monitor for reduced thyroid effect.

OBJECT DRUGS	PRECIPITANT DRUGS	
Tizanidine	**Enzyme Inhibitors:**	
(Zanaflex)	**Atazanavir** (Reyataz)	**Fluvoxamine** (Luvox)
	Cimetidine (Tagamet)	**Mexiletine** (Mexitil)
	Ciprofloxacin (Cipro)	**Tacrine** (Cognex)
	Enoxacin (Penetrex)	**Zileuton** (Zyflo)

COMMENTS: Potent CYP1A2 inhibitors such as fluvoxamine and ciprofloxacin can produce dramatic increases in tizanidine plasma concentrations; tizanidine toxicity is likely. Other CYP1A2 inhibitors would generally have less effect on tizanidine, but it would be prudent to avoid the combinations when possible.

MANAGEMENT CLASS 2: USE ONLY IF BENEFIT FELT TO OUTWEIGH RISK [CIPROFLOXACIN, ENOXACIN, FLUVOXAMINE]

- *Use Alternative:* Given the magnitude of the increase in tizanidine plasma concentrations, it would be prudent to avoid these combinations.
  Fluvoxamine: **Sertraline** (Zoloft), **fluoxetine** (Prozac), **venlafaxine** (Effexor), **paroxetine** (Paxil), **citalopram** (Celexa), and **escitalopram** (Lexapro) are not known to inhibit CYP1A2.
  Fluoroquinolones: **Gemifloxacin** (Factive), **levofloxacin** (Levaquin), **lomefloxacin** (Maxaquin), **moxifloxacin** (Avelox), **norfloxacin** (Noroxin), and **ofloxacin** (Floxin) appear to have little effect on CYP1A2.
- *Monitor:* If the combination is used, monitor for evidence of tizanidine toxicity such as hypotension and excessive CNS depression.

MANAGEMENT CLASS 3: ASSESS RISK AND TAKE ACTION IF NECESSARY [ATAZANAVIR, CIMETIDINE, MEXILETINE, TACRINE, ZILEUTON]

- *Consider Alternative:* If available, use a drug that is not an inhibitor of CYP1A2.
  Cimetidine: **Famotidine** (Pepcid), **nizatidine** (Axid), and **ranitidine** (Zantac) have no known effects on CYP1A2 activity.
- *Monitor:* If the combination is used, monitor for evidence of tizanidine toxicity such as hypotension and excessive CNS depression.

OBJECT DRUGS	PRECIPITANT DRUGS
Tyrosine Kinase Inhibitors (CYP3A4 Substrates):	**Antidepressants:**
Dasatinib (Sprycel)	**Fluvoxamine** (Luvox)
Erlotinib (Tarceva)	**Nefazodone**
Gefitinib (Iressa)	
Imatinib (Gleevec)	
Lapatinib (Tykerb)	
Nilotinib (Tasigna)	
Pazopanib (Votrient)	
Sorafenib (Nexavar)	
Sunitinib (Sutent)	

COMMENTS: Although data are limited, these antidepressants may increase the plasma levels of tyrosine kinase inhibitors. Toxicity including skin rashes, anemia, hemorrhage, and gastrointestinal symptoms could result. Assume that all CYP3A4 inhibitors interact until proven otherwise.

CLASS 3: ASSESS RISK & TAKE ACTION IF NECESSARY

- *Consider Alternative:*
  Antidepressants: **Citalopram** (Celexa), **desvenlafaxine** (Pristiq), **paroxetine** (Paxil), **sertraline** (Zoloft), and **venlafaxine** (Effexor) appear to have minimal effects on CYP3A4. **Fluoxetine** (Prozac) appears to be a weak inhibitor of CYP3A4.
- *Monitor:* Monitor for altered antineoplastic response if the CYP3A4 inhibitor is initiated, discontinued, or changed in dosage.

OBJECT DRUGS	PRECIPITANT DRUGS
Tyrosine Kinase Inhibitors	**Antimicrobials:**
(CYP3A4 Substrates):	**Clarithromycin** (Biaxin)
Dasatinib (Sprycel)	**Erythromycin** (E-Mycin)
Erlotinib (Tarceva)	**Fluconazole** (Diflucan)
Gefitinib (Iressa)	**Isoniazid** (INH)
Imatinib (Gleevec)	**Itraconazole** (Sporanox)
Lapatinib (Tykerb)	**Ketoconazole** (Nizoral)
Nilotinib (Tasigna)	**Posaconazole** (Noxafil)
Pazopanib (Votrient)	**Quinupristin** (Synercid)
Sorafenib (Nexavar)	**Telithromycin** (Ketek)
Sunitinib (Sutent)	**Troleandomycin** (TAO)
	Voriconazole (Vfend)

COMMENTS: Although data are limited, these antimicrobials may increase the plasma levels of tyrosine kinase inhibitors. Toxicity including skin rashes, anemia, hemorrhage, and gastrointestinal symptoms could result. Assume that all CYP3A4 inhibitors interact until proven otherwise.

CLASS 3: ASSESS RISK & TAKE ACTION IF NECESSARY

- *Consider Alternative*:
  Azole Antifungals: Fluconazole appears to be a less potent inhibitor of CYP3A4; but in larger doses it also inhibits CYP3A4. **Terbinafine** (Lamisil) does not appear to affect CYP3A4.
  Macrolide Antibiotics: **Azithromycin** (Zithromax) and **dirithromycin*** do not appear to inhibit CYP3A4 and are unlikely to interact. (*not available in US)
  Telithromycin: The use of **azithromycin** (Zithromax) or a quinolone antibiotic should be considered.
- *Monitor*: Monitor for altered antineoplastic response if the CYP3A4 inhibitor is initiated, discontinued, or changed in dosage.

OBJECT DRUGS	PRECIPITANT DRUGS	
Tyrosine Kinase Inhibitors **(CYP3A4 Substrates):** **Dasatinib** (Sprycel) **Erlotinib** (Tarceva) **Gefitinib** (Iressa) **Imatinib** (Gleevec) **Lapatinib** (Tykerb) **Nilotinib** (Tasigna) **Pazopanib** (Votrient) **Sorafenib** (Nexavar) **Sunitinib** (Sutent)	**Enzyme Inhibitors:** **Amiodarone** (Cordarone) **Amprenavir** (Agenerase) **Aprepitant** (Emend) **Atazanavir** (Reyataz) **Conivaptan** (Vaprisol) **Cyclosporine** (Neoral) **Darunavir** (Prezista) **Delavirdine** (Rescriptor)	**Diltiazem** (Cardizem) **Grapefruit** **Indinavir** (Crixivan) **Nelfinavir** (Viracept) **Ritonavir** (Norvir) **Saquinavir** (Invirase) **Verapamil** (Isoptin)

COMMENTS: Although data are limited, these enzyme inhibitors may increase the plasma levels of tyrosine kinase inhibitors. Toxicity including skin rashes, anemia, hemorrhage, and gastrointestinal symptoms could result. Assume that all CYP3A4 inhibitors interact until proven otherwise.

CLASS 3: ASSESS RISK & TAKE ACTION IF NECESSARY
- *Consider Alternative*:
  Calcium Channel Blockers: Calcium channel blockers other than diltiazem and verapamil are unlikely to inhibit the metabolism of these tyrosine kinase inhibitors.
  Grapefruit: Orange juice does not appear to inhibit CYP3A4.
- *Monitor*: Monitor for altered antineoplastic response if the CYP3A4 inhibitor is initiated, discontinued, or changed in dosage.

OBJECT DRUGS	PRECIPITANT DRUGS
Tyrosine Kinase Inhibitors **(CYP3A4 Substrates):** **Dasatinib** (Sprycel) **Erlotinib** (Tarceva) **Gefitinib** (Iressa) **Imatinib** (Gleevec) **Lapatinib** (Tykerb) **Nilotinib** (Tasigna) **Pazopanib** (Votrient) **Sorafenib** (Nexavar) **Sunitinib** (Sutent)	**Enzyme Inducers:** **Barbiturates** **Carbamazepine** (Tegretol) **Efavirenz** (Sustiva) **Nevirapine** (Viramune) **Oxcarbazepine** (Trileptal) **Phenytoin** (Dilantin) **Primidone** (Mysoline) **Rifabutin** (Mycobutin) **Rifampin** (Rifadin) **Rifapentine** (Priftin) **St. John's Wort**

COMMENTS: Although data are limited, these enzyme inducers may decrease the plasma levels of tyrosine kinase inhibitors. Reduction in the expected antineoplastic activity or resistance may occur.

CLASS 3: ASSESS RISK & TAKE ACTION IF NECESSARY
Monitor: Monitor for altered antineoplastic response if the CYP3A4 inducer is initiated, discontinued, or changed in dosage.

OBJECT DRUGS	PRECIPITANT DRUGS
Valproic Acid (Depakene)	**Carbapenem Antibiotics:**
	Ertapenem (Ivanz)
	Imipenem (Primaxin)
	Meropenem (Merrem)

COMMENTS: The administration of carbapenem antibiotics has been noted to markedly reduce the plasma concentrations of valproic acid. Reduction in seizure control may occur.

CLASS 3: ASSESS RISK & TAKE ACTION IF NECESSARY
- *Consider Alternative*: If possible, consider an alternative antibiotic to a carbapenem in patients taking valproic acid.
- *Monitor*: Monitor for altered valproic acid plasma concentrations and response if a carbapenem antibiotic is initiated, discontinued, or changed in dosage.

OBJECT DRUGS	PRECIPITANT DRUGS	
Vinca Alkaloids:	**Antimicrobials:**	
Vinblastine (Velban)	**Clarithromycin** (Biaxin)	**Posaconazole** (Noxafil)
Vincristine (Oncovin)	**Erythromycin** (E-Mycin)	**Quinupristin** (Synercid)
Vinorelbine (Navelbine)	**Fluconazole** (Diflucan)	**Telithromycin** (Ketek)
	Itraconazole (Sporanox)	**Troleandomycin** (TAO)
	Ketoconazole (Nizoral)	**Voriconazole** (Vfend)

COMMENTS: Vinca alkaloieds appear to be metabolized by CYP3A4, and several reports have described severe toxicity in patients receiving concurrent therapy with CYP3A4 inhibitors. Assume that all CYP3A4 inhibitors interact until proved otherwise. P-glycoprotein inhibition may also be involved in these interactions.

CLASS 2: USE ONLY IF BENEFIT FELT TO OUTWEIGH RISK
- *Use Alternative*:
  Azole Antifungals: Itraconazole and ketoconazole are potent inhibitors of CYP3A4; fluconazole appears weaker, but in larger doses it also inhibits CYP3A4. **Terbinafine** (Lamisil) does not appear to affect CYP3A4, and would not be expected to interact with vinca alkaloids.
  Macrolide Antibiotics: Unlike erythromycin, clarithromycin and troleandomycin, **azithromycin** (Zithromax) and **dirithromycin*** do not appear to inhibit CYP3A4. (*not available in US)
  Telithromycin: The use of **azithromycin** (Zithromax) or a quinolone antibiotic should be considered.
- *Monitor*: Monitor for toxicity from vincristine (primarily peripheral neuropathy symptoms: paresthesias, neuritic pain, muscle pain, constipation sometimes progressing to paralytic ileus) or vinblastine and vinorelbine (primarily bone marrow suppression).

OBJECT DRUGS	PRECIPITANT DRUGS
Vinca Alkaloids:	**Calcium Channel Blockers:**
Vinblastine (Velban)	**Diltiazem** (Cardizem)
Vincristine (Oncovin)	**Nicardipine** (Cardene)
Vinorelbine (Navelbine)	**Nifedipine** (Procardia)
	Verapamil (Isoptin)

COMMENTS: Vina alkaloids appear to be metabolized by CYP3A4 and several reports have described severe vincristine toxicity in patients receiving CYP3A4 inhibitors such as verapamil. P-glycoprotein inhibition may also be involved in these interactions.

CLASS 2: USE ONLY IF BENEFIT FELT TO OUTWEIGH RISK
- *Use Alternative*: Use an alternative to the enzyme inhibitor if possible.
  Calcium channel blockers: Calcium channel blockers other than diltiazem, nicardipine, nifedipine, and verapamil are unlikely to inhibit the metabolism of vinca alkaloids.
- *Monitor*: Monitor for toxicity from vincristine (primarily peripheral neuropathy symptoms: paresthesias, neuritic pain, muscle pain, constipation sometimes progressing to paralytic ileus) or vinblastine and vinorelbine (primarily bone marrow suppression).

OBJECT DRUGS	PRECIPITANT DRUGS	
Vinca Alkaloids:	**Enzyme Inhibitors:**	
Vinblastine (Velban)	**Amiodarone** (Cordarone)	**Fluvoxamine** (Luvox)
Vincristine (Oncovin)	**Amprenavir** (Agenerase)	**Grapefruit**
Vinorelbine (Navelbine)	**Aprepitant** (Emend)	**Indinavir** (Crixivan)
	Atazanavir (Reyataz)	**Nefazodone**
	Conivaptan (Vaprisol)	**Nelfinavir** (Viracept)
	Cyclosporine (Neoral)	**Ritonavir** (Norvir)
	Darunavir (Prezista)	**Saquinavir** (Invirase)
	Delavirdine (Rescriptor)	

COMMENTS: Vinca alkaloids appear to be metabolized by CYP3A4 and several reports have described severe vincristine toxicity in patients receiving CYP3A4 inhibitors. P-glycoprotein inhibition may also be involved in these interactions.

CLASS 2: USE ONLY IF BENEFIT FELT TO OUTWEIGH RISK
- *Use Alternative*: Use an alternative to the enzyme inhibitor if possible.
  Antidepressants: **Sertraline** (Zoloft), **citalopram** (Celexa), **escitalopram** (Lexapro), **venlafaxine** (Effexor), and **paroxetine** (Paxil) appear less likely to inhibit CYP3A4. **Fluoxetine** (Prozac) appears to be only a weak inhibitor of CYP3A4.
  Grapefruit: Orange juice does not appear to inhibit CYP3A4.
- *Monitor*: Monitor for toxicity from vincristine (primarily peripheral neuropathy symptoms: paresthesias, neuritic pain, muscle pain, constipation sometimes progressing to paralytic ileus) or vinblastine and vinorelbine (primarily bone marrow suppression).

OBJECT DRUGS	PRECIPITANT DRUGS	
Zidovudine (Retrovir)	**Enzyme Inducers:**	
	Barbiturates	**Primidone** (Mysoline)
	Carbamazepine (Tegretol)	**Rifabutin** (Mycobutin)
	Efavirenz (Sustiva)	**Rifampin** (Rifadin)
	Nevirapine (Viramune)	**Rifapentine** (Priftin)
	Oxcarbazepine (Trileptal)	**St. John's Wort**
	Phenytoin (Dilantin)	

COMMENTS: Enzyme inducers such as rifampin and rifabutin may enhance zidovudine metabolism, thus reducing its effect. Little is known regarding the effect of other enzyme inducers on zidovudine, but consider the possibility of a similar interaction.

CLASS 3: ASSESS RISK & TAKE ACTION IF NECESSARY

- *Consider Alternative:* If available, use a drug that is not an enzyme inducer. St. John's Wort: Given the limited evidence of efficacy, St. John's Wort should generally be avoided in patients taking zidovudine.
- *Monitor:* Zidovudine dose may need to be adjusted if enzyme inducer therapy is initiated or discontinued. Keep in mind that enzyme induction is usually gradual and may take days to weeks for onset and offset, depending on the specific inducer.

OBJECT DRUGS	PRECIPITANT DRUGS
Zidovudine (Retrovir)	**Glucuronidation Inhibitors:**
	Probenecid (Benemid)
	Trimethoprim (Bactrim)
	Valproic acid (Depakene)

COMMENTS: Drugs that can inhibit glucuronidation such as probenecid, trimethoprim, and valproic acid may increase zidovudine serum concentrations, probably by inhibition of hepatic metabolism (reduced renal excretion may also be involved).

CLASS 3: ASSESS RISK & TAKE ACTION IF NECESSARY

- *Consider Alternative:* If possible use an alternative to the glucuronidation inhibitor. Some have recommended use of an alternative to the zidovudine that is not metabolized by glucuronidation. In one case substitution of **stavudine** (Zerit) for zidovudine was successful.
- *Monitor:* Zidovudine dose may need to be adjusted if these drugs are initiated, discontinued or changed in dosage. Watch for anemia in patients receiving zidovudine and valproic acid.

Effect of Other Antibiotics on Warfarin

It is important to note that both infection and inflammation can alter warfarin metabolism by increasing the production of cytokines. Several cytokines have been noted to reduce the activity of CYP2C9, the enzyme primarily responsible for the metabolism of S-warfarin. When one considers the effect of cytokines combined with possible reduced intake of vitamin K during acute illness and fever-induced increase in catabolism of clotting factors, it is not unexpected that patients requiring antibiotics may have increased warfarin effect. This change in warfarin response may occur at the same time as antibiotic administration, but be unrelated to the administration of the antibiotic.

Antibiotic	Effect on Warfarin
Cephalosporins (NMTT side chain)	Cephalosporins with an NMTT side chain such as **cefoperazone** (Cefobid), **cefamandole** (Mandol), **cefotetan** (Cefotan), and **moxalactam** (Moxam) have been associated with hypoprothrombinemia.
Macrolides and Ketolides	**Erythromycin** produces small increases in warfarin response in most people but occasionally marked increases occur. **Clarithromycin** (Biaxin) and **telithromycin** (Ketek), like erythromycin, have been reported to increase warfarin effect. Isolated cases of increased warfarin effect reported with **azithromycin** (Zithromax) but a causal relationship is not established.
Penicillins, (Extended Spectrum)	Occasionally, IV **ticarcillin** (Ticar) and to a lesser extent **mezlocillin** (Mezlin) and **piperacillin** (Pipracil) produce coagulation disorders (prolonged bleeding or increased INR).
Penicillin G	Isolated cases of increased warfarin effect reported with high dose IV penicillin G; clinical importance is not known.
Quinolones	Isolated cases of increased warfarin effect reported with quinolones such as **ciprofloxacin** (Cipro), **levofloxacin** (Levaquin), **moxifloxacin** (Avelox), **nalidixic acid** (NegGram), **norfloxacin** (Noroxin), and **ofloxacin** (Floxin), but a causal relationship is not clear; most quinolones do not appear to affect warfarin pharmacokinetics or hypoprothrombinemia.
Tetracyclines	Isolated cases of increased warfarin effect with various tetracyclines; clinical importance not established.

Drug Interactions with Drugs that Increase QTc Intervals

A variety of drugs can affect the electrical activity of cardiac muscle. Normal cardiac contraction requires a rapid depolarization of the muscle followed by a slower repolarization. Repolarization is primarily accomplished by potassium efflux from the cell. Drugs can delay repolarization and prolong the cardiac action potential by blocking this potassium efflux. The delayed repolarization can be seen on the ECG as a prolongation of the QTc interval. Delayed repolarization enables an inward flow of calcium and premature depolarization. Early afterdepolarizations can trigger arrhythmias including torsades de pointes.

Some antiarrhythmic drugs such as amiodarone, procainamide, quinidine, sotalol, and dofetilide prolong repolarization as part of their therapeutic action and do so at therapeutic plasma concentrations. The incidence of torsades de pointes with these drugs has been noted to be <5 per 100 patients. Other drugs, not classified as antiarrhythmic agents, e.g., phenothiazines, and some antibiotics, also slow repolarization by affecting potassium efflux. At plasma concentrations above usual therapeutic levels, these drugs may also produce arrhythmias. The risk of torsades de pointes is much less likely with these agents; perhaps 1 per 100,000 patients, although the exact incidence is not known.

Normal QTc duration is less than 440ms while QTc durations exceeding 500ms are more frequently associated with arrhythmias. QTc may vary by as much as 50 - 75ms over a 24 hour period in normal individuals. There is no agreement on the degree of QTc prolongation that is considered safe. Some believe no amount of increase is safe while others are not concerned with increases <35ms provided normal limits are not exceeded. Several factors including, hypokalemia, hypomagnesemia, bradycardia, hypertrophy, heart failure, and female gender predispose patients to increased clinical risk from prolonged QTc intervals. Although a prolonged QTc does not often lead to arrhythmias, patients with large QTc prolongations (e.g.,> 60ms above baseline) may be at the greatest risk to develop arrhythmias including torsades de pointes.

The chart on page 116 categorizes drugs that have been noted to increase the QTc interval. They are grouped based on their ability to alter the QTc at therapeutic or elevated plasma concentrations. Data are very limited regarding the ability of these drugs to induce arrhythmias when used alone or in combination. However, caution should be used when combinations of these agents are prescribed, particularly if the combination results in a pharmacokinetic interaction. Refer to the Table on page 117 to identify combinations with potential pharmacokinetic interactions and those combinations that are limited to pharmacodynamic interactions and thus less likely to produce an arrhythmia. Consider substituting related drugs that do not affect the QTc interval as alternatives to one of the potentially interacting drugs. For example, SSRI antidepressants that do not inhibit CYP450 enzymes could be used in place of tricyclic antidepressants, or a quinolone without potential cardiac effects could be substituted for a quinolone reported to prolong the QTc interval.

Management Classes for Prolonged QTc Interval Drug Interactions
(For Use With Drug Charts on Next Page)

Management Class 1: Avoid Combination.

a. Any two drugs from Column I. (e.g., Dofetilide + Qunidine)

b. A drug from Column I plus a drug from Column II that also have a pharmacokinetic interaction. (e.g., Quinidine + Thioridazine)

Management Class 2: Use only if Benefit Felt to Outweigh Risk.

a. A drug from Column I plus a drug from Column II that *do not* have a pharmacokinetic interaction (pharmacodynamic interaction only). (e.g., Procainamide + Haloperidol)

b. Any two drugs from Column II that *also* have a pharmacokinetic interaction. (e.g., Cisapride + Erythromycin)

c. Any drug from Column I plus a drug that produces a pharmacokinetic interaction. (e.g., Quinidine + Ketoconazole)

Management Class 3: Assess risk and take action if necessary.

a. Any two drugs from Column II that *do not* have a pharmacokinetic interaction (pharmacodynamic interaction only). (e.g., Clozapine + Ziprasidone)

b. A drug from Column II plus a drug that inhibits its metabolism. (e.g., Amitriptyline + Propoxyphene)

Note: Class 2 and 3 drug combinations should be administered only with ECG monitoring for potential changes in QTc interval; when appropriate, monitor also plasma concentration of the antiarrhythmic.

Drugs Reported to Prolong the QTc Interval[a]

Column I	Column II
Drugs that prolong the QTc interval at therapeutic concentrations.	Drugs that may produce clinically relevant prolongation of the QTc interval at elevated concentrations.
Amiodarone (Cordarone)	Amitriptyline (Elavil)[b]
Disopyramide (Norpace)	Arsenic trioxide (Trisenox)
Dofetilide (Tikosyn)	Bepridil (Vascor)
Dronedarone (Multaq)	Chloroquine (Aralen)
Ibutilide (Covert)	Chlorpromazine (Thorazine)
Lapatinib (Tykerb)	Cisapride (Propulsid)
Procainamide (Procanbid)	Clarithromycin (Biaxin)
N-acetylprocainamide	Clomipramine (Anafranil)[b]
Quinidine (Quinidex)	Clozapine (Clozaril)
Sotalol (Betapace)	Desipramine (Norpramin)
	Dolasetron (Anzemet)
	Droperidol (Inapsine)
	Erythromycin (E-Mycin)
	Gatifloxacin (Tequin)
	Haloperidol (Haldol)
	Levofloxacin (Levaquin)
	Levomethadyl (Orlaam)
	Mefloquine (Lariam)
	Mesoridazine (Serentil)
	Methadone
	Moxifloxacin (Avelox)
	Nilotinib (Tasigna)
	Ondansetron (Zofran)
	Pimozide (Orap)
	Ranolazine (Ranexa)
	Sumatriptan (Imitrex)
	Thioridazine (Mellaril)
	Ziprasidone (Geodon)
	Zolmitriptan (Zomig)

a. Note that the lists are not exhaustive, nor should a drug's listing in a specific column be considered absolute. As additional data become available, drug listings are subject to change. Some drugs have profound effects on QTc while others produce only minor changes, particularly in the absence of predisposing factors.

b. Widens the QRS interval.

Drugs Reported to Prolong QTc Intervals:
Known Substrates and Inhibitors of CYP2D6 and CYP3A4

CYP Enzyme	Substrates	Inhibitors[c]
CYP2D6	Amitriptyline[a] Chlorpromazine Clomipramine[a] Desipramine Haloperidol Propafenone Risperidone[a] Thioridazine	Amiodarone Dronedarone Haloperidol Quinidine Propafenone Thioridazine
CYP3A4	Amiodarone Amitriptyline Bepridil Cisapride Clomipramine Dofetilide[b] Dronedarone Droperidol Lapatinib Levomethadyl Nilotinib Ondansetron Pimozide Quinidine Ranolazine Ziprasidone[d]	Amiodarone Clarithromycin Dronedarone Erythromycin

a. CYP2D6 is the primary pathway

b. Dofetilide has about 70% renal elimination

c. Other drugs that inhibit CYP2D6 or CYP3A4 may also interact. See the Table Cytochrome P450 Enzymes and Transporters for more potential inhibitors of the substrates listed above.

d. Ziprasidone is about 33% metabolized by CYP3A4; aldehyde oxidase metabolizes most of the remainder.

Genetic Polymorphisms of Cytochrome P450 Enzymes

The pharmacogenetics of drug-metabolizing enzymes contributes to the variability observed between patients receiving the same two interacting drugs at the same doses. Differences in the genetic makeup of enzymes (genotype) can lead to altered patient responses including toxicity or lack of efficacy (phenotype). The table below lists common CYP450 enzymes known to have different genotypes. Differing genotypes result in patients that are often referred to as extensive or poor metabolizers of drugs that are substrates for a specific cytochrome P450 enzyme. Poor metabolizers (PMs) will accumulate more of the parent drug. However, since their ability to metabolize the drug is limited, they are protected from other drugs that may inhibit the enzyme. Extensive metabolizers (EMs) will have greater enzyme activity and lower concentrations of the parent drug, but tend to be very sensitive to other drugs that inhibit the enzyme. EMs often demonstrate very large reductions in the metabolism of object drugs when an inhibitor is coadministered and are at greater risk of developing an adverse outcome from a drug interaction. Polymorphisms are clinically most important for drugs with a narrow therapeutic range and when the polymorphic pathway is responsible for a major portion of the drug's metabolism.

Enzyme	Frequency of PMs	Examples of drugs affected
CYP2C9	6-8%	Glyburide, Glipizide, Warfarin, Phenytoin
CYP2C19	3-5% Caucasians 12-23% Asians	Diazepam, Omeprazole, Pantoprazole
CYP2D6[a]	6-10% Caucasians[b] 3-6% Mexican Americans 2-5% African Americans 1% Asians[c]	Codeine, Imipramine, Propafenone, Metoprolol
CYP3A4/5	Under Study	Numerous (probably half of all drugs are metabolized by CYP3A4/5

a. Note that *increased* CYP2D6 activity may also occur. Approximate prevalence of "Ultrarapid" CYP2D6 metabolizers: Finns and Danes 1%; North Americans (white) 4%; Greeks 10%; Portuguese 10%; Saudis 20%; Ethiopians 30%. Such people may have low concentrations of CYP2D6 substrates, and may also develop morphine toxicity when given the pro-drug codeine.

b. Most Caucasians are "Extensive Metabolizers" (EMs) of CYP2D6.

c. Roughly half of Asians are "Intermediate Metabolizers" of CYP2D6, meaning that they have CYP2D6 activity that is in between "Poor Metabolizers" and "Rapid Metabolizers."

Drug Interactions with Herbal Products

There has been increasing attention to the interactions of medications with herbal products, and some herbal drug interactions are relatively well documented. For example, ephedrine is an indirect-acting sympathomimetic that may result in acute hypertension when combined with MAO inhibitors. Kava and valerian have well-documented sedative properties, and may have additive effects with other CNS depressant drugs. St. John's wort is an inducer of CYP3A4, and probably also induces CYP2C9 and P-glycoprotein. It appears to interact with a variety of drugs that are substrates for these isozymes and transporters.

Other purported drug interactions of herbal products are not as well documented, and are often based on case reports in which a causal relationship is tentative. For example the purported ability of many herbal products to increase the risk of bleeding in patients receiving warfarin is based primarily on isolated case reports and in vitro/animal studies. Several herbal products reportedly inhibit platelet function, thereby increasing the risk of bleeding in patients on oral anticoagulants, but there is very little supporting clinical evidence. Many other suspected herbal-drug interactions are based on similarly inadequate clinical information.

Moreover, prevention of adverse drug-herbal interactions is hampered by several other factors. Herbal medications are usually not standardized, so different herbal brands may interact differently with other medications due to different amounts of active ingredient or additional ingredients not on the label (and in some cases no active ingredients at all). Moreover, different lots of the same brand may vary substantially as to content as well. Herbal medications are often absent from computerized drug interaction screening systems, so it is important to educate patients to keep their health professionals informed of all alternative medications. **Note**: Some herbal drug interactions are included in the preceding monographs, and can be found by consulting the index.

Object Drugs	Precipitant Drugs

Alprazolam (Xanax) · **St. John's Wort**
St. John's wort substantially reduces alprazolam plasma concentrations, and would be expected to reduce alprazolam response. Other benzodiazepines that are CYP3A4 substrates (e.g., midazolam, triazolam) may be similarly affected.

Amygdalin · **Vitamin C**
A cancer patient on vitamin C 4800 mg/day developed cyanide toxicity with seizures and lactic acidosis soon after taking one dose of amygdalin, possibly through increased conversion of amygdalin to cyanide. Although more data are

needed, the severity of the reaction suggests that patients taking amygdalin avoid high dose vitamin C.

CNS Depressants: **Kava**
Alcohol
Barbiturates
Benzodiazepines
Opiates
Kava is a central nervous system depressant, and may have additive depressant effects with other CNS depressants. Monitor patient for evidence of excessive CNS depression.

CNS Depressants: **Valerian**
Alcohol
Barbiturates
Benzodiazepines
Opiates
Valerain is a central nervous system depressant, and may have additive depressant effects with other CNS depressants. Monitor patient for evidence of excessive CNS depression.

Contraceptives, Oral   **St. John's Wort**
See monograph on page 60.

Cyclosporine (Neoral)   **Echinacea**
Echinacea purportedly may reduce the efficacy of cyclosporine and other immunosuppressants. This is based on theoretical considerations, however, and the clinical importance of this purported interaction is unknown.

Cyclosporine (Neoral)   **St. John's Wort**
See monograph on page 74.

Cyclosporine (Neoral)   **Zinc**
Zinc, acting as an "immunostimulant", purportedly may reduce the efficacy of cyclosporine and other immunosuppressants. This is based on theoretical considerations, however, and the clinical importance of this purported interaction is unknown.

Digoxin (Lanoxin)   **Ginseng**
A case of increased digoxin serum concentrations following Siberian ginseng has been reported, possibly due to interference with digoxin assay. The clinical importance of this purported interaction is not established, but one should monitor for altered digoxin concentrations and response when any herbal product is added (many herbal products reportedly contain digoxin-like substances).

Digoxin (Lanoxin)　　　　　　　　　**St. John's Wort**
Pharmacokinetic study in healthy subjects suggest that St. John's wort may modestly reduce digoxin serum concentrations, probably due to St. John's wort-induced increase in P-glycoprotein activity. The extent to which this interaction would result in reduced digoxin efficacy is not known. Monitor patients for reduced digoxin response and digoxin serum concentrations.

Erlotinib (Tarceva)　　　　　　　　　**St. John's Wort**
See monograph on page 109.

Felodipine (Plendil)　　　　　　　　　**Peppermint Oil**
Peppermint oil moderately increased felodipine plasma concentrations, but the clinical importance of this interaction is not established.

Fexofenadine (Allegra)　　　　　　　　**St. John's Wort**
St. John's wort can substantially reduce the plasma concentration of fexofenadine. Avoid concurrent use.

Glipizide (Glucotrol)　　　　　　　　　**St. John's Wort**
St. John's wort can reduce the plasma concentration of glipizide. St. John's wort should generally be avoided in patients taking glipizide.

Ibuprofen (Advil, Motrin)　　　　　　　**St. John's Wort**
St. John's wort can reduce the plasma concentration of ibuprofen. St. John's wort should generally be avoided in patients taking ibuprofen.

Imatinib (Gleevec)　　　　　　　　　　**St. John's Wort**
See monograph on page 109.

Indinavir (Crixivan)　　　　　　　　　**St. John's Wort**
See monograph on page 90.

Irinotecan (Camptosar)　　　　　　　　**St. John's Wort**
St. John's wort can substantially reduce irinotecan plasma concentrations; St. John's wort should generally be avoided in patients on irinotecan.

Levodopa　　　　　　　　　　　　　　**Kava**
A patient with Parkinson's disease treated with levodopa had increased "off" periods during kava use. Confirmation is needed, but monitor for altered efficacy of antiparkinson drugs if kava is used.

Loperamide (Imodium)　　　　　　　　　**St. John's Wort**
A patient on concurrent loperamide, St. John's wort and valerian developed

delirium, but a causal relationship was not established.

MAO Inhibitors   **Ephedrine**
Severe hypertensive reactions are likely, and the combination is contraindicated.

MAO Inhibitors   **Ginseng**
The use of ginseng has been associated with isolated cases of toxicity (e.g., headache, insomnia, irritability, tremor) in patients receiving phenelzine (Nardil), but a causal relationship was not established. Although the potential interaction is poorly documented, given the lack of evidence of ginseng efficacy, the combination would best be avoided. If the combination is used the patient should be carefully monitored for adverse effects.

Melatonin   **Fluvoxamine (Luvox)**
Based on a pharmacokinetic study in healthy subjects, fluvoxamine may produce a marked increase in melatonin serum concentrations. Although the clinical importance of this effect is not established, one should watch for evidence of excessive melatonin effect if the combination is used.

Midazolam (Versed)   **Echinacea**
In healthy subjects echinacea increased oral midazolam plasma concentrations and decreased intravenous midazolam plasma concentrations. The clinical importance of these interactions is not established.

Nevirapine (Viramune)   **St. John's Wort**
In five HIV positive patients, the use of St. John's wort was associated with reduced nevirapine plasma concentrations compared with the same patients without St. John's wort. A database of 176 patients on nevirapine also suggested reduced nevirapine plasma concentrations with St. John's wort. Patients on nevirapine should probably avoid taking St. John's wort.

Nifedipine (Procardia)   **Melatonin**
Hypertensive patients stabilized on nifedipine developed increased blood pressure after the use of melatonin. The clinical importance of this effect is not established.

NSAIDs   **Ginkgo Biloba**
Ginkgo and NSAIDS purportedly may display additive inhibitory effects on platelet function, but the clinical importance of this effect is unknown.

Omeprazole (Prilosec)   **St. John's Wort**
In healthy subjects St. John's wort reduced omeprazole plasma concentrations by about 40%. Although the clinical importance of this effect is not established, one should be alert for reduced omeprazole effect.

Rosuvastatin (Crestor)   **Baicalin**

Baicalin may reduce rosuvastatin plasma concentrations, probably by inducing OATP. Baicalin is found in seferal Chinese herbal products.

Saquinavir (Invirase)   **Garlic**

Garlic capsules substantially reduced saquinavir serum concentrations in healthy subjects. Although confirmation is needed, it would be prudent to monitor for reduced saquinavir effect if garlic is used concurrently. In another study, garlic did not affect ritonavir pharmacokinetics in healthy subjects.

Selective Serotonin Reuptake   **St. John's Wort**
Inhibitors (SSRIs)

St. John's wort has reportedly produced serotonin syndrome when given to patients receiving SSRIs. The symptoms reported, however, have not been the classic findings of serotonin syndrome. Nonetheless, one should watch for evidence of serotonin syndrome if the combination is used. Serotonin syndrome can result in neurotoxicity (myoclonus, tremors, rigidity, incoordination, hyperreflexia, seizures, coma), psychiatric symptoms (agitation, confusion, hypomania, restlessness), and autonomic dysfunction (fever, sweating, tachycardia, hypertension).

Theophylline   **St. John's Wort**

See monograph on page 102.

Verapamil   **St. John's Wort**

See monograph on page 51.

Voriconazole (Vfend)   **St. John's Wort**

St. John's wort reduced the concentration of voriconazole by over 50%. Avoid concurrent use.

Warfarin (Coumadin)   **Boldo-Fenugreek**

A patient stabilized on warfarin developed an increased INR after starting a herbal product containing boldo-fenugreek. A positive dechallenge and rechallenge suggests a causal relationship. If boldo-fenugreek is used with warfarin, monitor for bleeding and changes in INR.

Warfarin (Coumadin)   **Coenzyme Q10**

Several cases have been reported of reduced hypoprothrombinemic response in patients receiving warfarin who received coenzyme Q10 concomitantly. Although a causal relationship was not established, the combination would be best avoided; if it is used the patient should be carefully monitored for changes in INR.

Warfarin (Coumadin)   **Cranberry**

Cranberry juice or sauce has been implicated in several cases of marked INR increases in patients on warfarin; at least two cases were fatal. In a randomized crossover trial in 12 healthy subjects cranberry concentrate increased warfarin INR by 30%, but did not affect warfarin pharmacokinetics. It would be prudent to advise patients on warfarin to avoid large amounts of cranberry juice or sauce. If cranberry is ingested, monitor the INR.

Warfarin (Coumadin)   **Danshen**

Danshen has been associated with several cases of increased hypoprothrombinemic response and bleeding in patients receiving warfarin. Although a causal relationship has not been conclusively established, the combination would be best avoided. If the combination is used, the patient should be carefully monitored for increased INR and bleeding.

Warfarin (Coumadin)   **Dong Quai**

Dong quai has been associated with isolated cases of increased hypoprothrombinemic response in patients on warfarin. Dong quai purportedly also inhibits platelet function. Although the clinical importance of this effect is unknown, as with any drug added to warfarin, the patient should be monitored for evidence of bleeding and changes in INR.

Warfarin (Coumadin)   **Feverfew**

Feverfew purportedly may increase the risk of bleeding in patients on warfarin due to inhibition of platelet function, but the clinical importance of this effect is unknown. As with any drug added to warfarin, the patient should be monitored for evidence of bleeding and changes in INR.

Warfarin (Coumadin)   **Garlic**

Garlic supplements purportedly increase the risk of bleeding due to inhibition of platelet function, but the clinical importance of this effect is unknown. In a crossover study of healthy subjects, garlic did not affect the INR response to warfarin. Pending more information, patients should be monitored for evidence of bleeding and changes in INR if garlic products are used. There is no evidence that garlic in food affects the bleeding risk in patients on warfarin.

Warfarin (Coumadin)   **Ginger**

Ginger purportedly may increase the risk of bleeding due to inhibition of platelet function, but the clinical importance of this effect is unknown. Study in healthy subjects suggests that ginger dies not affect warfarin pharmacokinetics. If the combination is used, patients should be monitored for evidence of bleeding and changes in INR.

Warfarin (Coumadin)   **Ginkgo Biloba**

Ginkgo has been associated with isolated cases of severe bleeding in patients receiving warfarin or aspirin, but a causal relationship was not established. Some evidence suggests that ginkgo inhibits platelet function, an effect that would not be reflected in an increased INR. Although more evidence is needed, it would be prudent to avoid the combination.

Warfarin (Coumadin)   **Ginseng**

Isolated case reports and study in healthy subjects suggest that ginseng can reduce the effect of warfarin. Another study found no effect of ginseng, but it involved fewer days of ginseng exposure. Given the lack of evidence of ginseng efficacy, the combination should generally be avoided. If the combination is used, patients should be carefully monitored for altered INR.

Warfarin (Coumadin)   **Glucosamine**

A number of case reports suggest that glucosamine can increase the effect of warfarin, but most of the cases have been spontaneous reports to adverse reaction database agencies. A causal relationship is not established. Pending additional information, monitored for altered INR if the combination is used.

Warfarin (Coumadin)   **Green Tea**

A patient on warfarin developed inhibition of the hypoprothrombinemic response after consuming large amounts of green tea daily (up to 1 gallon). Although a causal relationship was not established, until more information is available it would be prudent to advise patients on warfarin to avoid large amounts of green tea.

Warfarin (Coumadin)   **Pomegranate Juice**

Isolated cases of increased warfarin response have been reported; more study is needed to establish the clinical importance.

Warfarin (Coumadin)   **Quilinggao**

A patient stabilized on warfarin developed bleeding and an elevated INR after taking a Chinese herbal product containing quilinggao. Another brand of quilinggao later produced a similar effect. If quilinggao is used with warfarin, monitor for bleeding and changes in INR.

Warfarin (Coumadin)   **St. John's Wort**

See monograph on page 27.

INDEX

<u>Underline</u> = Class 1; *Italic* = Class 2;   Roman = Class 3

<u>Underline</u> = Class 1;   *Italic* = Class 2;   Roman = Class 3

<u>Underline</u> = Class 1;   *Italic* = Class 2;   Roman = Class 3

Barbiturates 90
Bepridil 53
Bosentan 90
Buspirone 43
Carbamazepine 55,90
Clarithromycin 78
Clonazepam 43
Clorazepate 43
Conivaptan 92
Corticosteroids 63
Cyclosporine, 75,92
Darunavir 92
Dasatinib 109
Delavirdine 92
Diazepam 43
Diltiazem 53,92
Disopyramide 24
Dronedarone 24
Efavirenz 90
Eplerenone 68
Ergot Alkaloids 70
Erlotinib 109
Erythromycin 90
Estazolam 43
Felodipine 53
Fentanyl 83
Fluconazole 90
Flurazepam 43
Fluvoxamine 91
Gefitinib 109
Grapefruit 92
Halazepam 43
Imatinib 109
Indinavir 92
Isradipine 53
Itraconazole 90
Ketoconazole 90
Lapatinib 109
Lopinavir 92
Lovastatin 73
Methadone 83
Midazolam 43
Nateglinide 38
Nefazodone 91
Nelfinavir 92
Nevirapine 90
Nicardipine 53

Nifedipine 53
Nilotinib 109
Nimodipine 53
Nisoldipine 53
Nitrendipine 53
Oxcarbazepine 90
Oxycodone 83
Pazopanib 109
Phenytoin 90
<u>Pimozide</u> 88
Pioglitazone 38
Posaconazole 90
Prazepam 43
Primidone 77
Quetiapine 94
Quinidine 24
Quinupristin 90
Ranolazine 96
Repaglinide 38
Rifabutin 90,98
Rifampin 90
Rifapentine 90
Ritonavir 92
Saquinavir 92
Saxagliptin 38
Sildenafil 100
Simvastatin 73
Sirolimus 75
Sorafenib 109
St. John's Wort 90
Sufentanil 83
Sunitinib 109
Tacrolimus 75
Tadalafil 100
Telithromycin 90
Tipranavir 92
Triazolam 43
Troleandomycin 90
Vardenafil 100
Verapamil 53,92
Vinblastine 111
Vincristine 111
Vinorelbine 111
Voriconazole 90
Amygdalin. See Herbal
  Interaction chart
Anafranil. See Clomipramine

Angiotensin Converting
  Enzyme Inhibitors. See
  ACE Inhibitors
Angiotensin Receptor
  Blockers
  Aspirin 39
  Diclofenac 39
  Diflunisal 39
  Etodolac 39
  Fenoprofen 39
  Flurbiprofen 39
  Ibuprofen 39
  Indomethacin 39
  Ketoprofen 39
  Ketorolac 39
  Lithium 77
  Meclofenamate 39
  Mefenamic acid 39
  Meloxicam 39
  Nabumetone 39
  Naproxen 39
  Oxaprozin 39
  Sulindac 39
  Tolmetin 39
Androgens
  Acenocoumarol 31
  Cyclosporine 75
  Sirolimus 75
  Tacrolimus 75
  Warfarin 31
Ansaid. See Flurbiprofen
Antabuse. See Disulfiram
Antacids
  Cefditoren 56
  Cefpodoxime 56
  Cefuroxime 56
  Ciprofloxacin 95
  Enoxacin 95
  Gemifloxacin 95
  Glipizide 38
  Glyburide 38
  Itraconazole 48
  Ketoconazole 48
  Levofloxacin 95
  Lomefloxacin 95
  Moxifloxacin 95
  Mycophenolate 85

<u>Underline</u> = Class 1;   *Italic* = Class 2;   Roman = Class 3

Itraconazole 44
Ketoconazole 44
Nefazodone 45
Nelfinavir 45
Nevirapine 43
Oxcarbazepine 43
Paroxetine 45
Phenytoin 43
Posaconazole 44
Primidone 43
Propafenone 46
Propoxyphene 46
Quinidine 46
Quinupristin 44
Rifabutin 43
Rifampin 43
Rifapentine 43
Ritonavir 45,46
Saquinavir 45
St. John's wort 43
Telithromycin 44
Terbinafine 46
Thioridazine 46
Troleandomycin 44
Verapamil 45
Voriconazole 44
Aristocort. See
 Triamcinolone
Asendin. See Antidepressants, tricyclic
Aspirin
 Acenocoumarol 26
 ACE Inhibitors 39
 Angiotensin Receptor
  Blockers 39
 Ibuprofen 46
 Methotrexate 84
 Phenprocoumon 26
 Pralatrexate 84
 Warfarin 26
Atacand. See Angiotensin
 Receptor Blockers
Atazanavir
 Alfuzosin 22
 Alprazolam 43
 Alfentanil 83
 Amiodarone 24,92

Amlodipine 53
Amprenavir 92
Antidepressants,
 tricyclic 34
Aprepitant 92
Aripiprazole 45
Atorvastatin 73
Barbiturates 90
Bepridil 53
Bosentan 90
Buspirone 43
Carbamazepine 55,90
Clarithromycin 90
Clonazepam 43
Clorazepate 43
Clozapine 57
Colchicine 60
Conivaptan 92
Corticosteroids 63
Cyclosporine 75,92
Darunavir 92
Dasatinib 109
Delavirdine 92
Diazepam 43
Diltiazem 53,79
Disopyramide 24
Dronedarone 24
Efavirenz 90
Eplerenone 68
Ergot Alkaloids 70
Erlotinib 109
Erythromycin 90
Estazolam 43
Felodipine 53
Fentanyl 83
Fluconazole 90
Flurazepam 43
Fluvoxamine 91
Gefitinib 109
Grapefruit 92
Halazepam 43
Imatinib 109
Indinavir 92
Isradipine 53
Itraconazole 90
Ketoconazole 90
Lapatinib 109

Lopinavir 92
Lovastatin 73
Methadone 83
Midazolam 43
Nateglinide 38
Nefazodone 91
Nelfinavir 92
Nevirapine 90
Nicardipine 53
Nifedipine 53
Nilotinib 109
Nimodipine 53
Nisoldipine 53
Nitrendipine 53
Olanzapine 57
Oxcarbazepine 90
Oxycodone 83
Pazopanib 109
Phenytoin 90
Pimozide 88
Pioglitazone 38
Posaconazole 90
Prazepam 43
Primidone 90
Quetiapine 94
Quinidine 24
Quinupristin 90
Ranolazine 96
Repaglinide 38
Rifabutin 90,98
Rifampin 90
Rifapentine 90
Ritonavir 92
Saquinavir 92
Saxagliptin 38
Sildenafil 100
Simvastatin 73
Sirolimus 75
Sorafenib 109
St. John's Wort 90
Sufentanil 83
Sunitinib 109
Tacrolimus 83
Tadalafil 100
Telithromycin 90
Theophylline 103
Tipranavir 92

Underline = Class 1;   *Italic* = Class 2;   Roman = Class 3

Underline = Class 1;   *Italic* = Class 2;   Roman = Class 3

<u>Underline</u> = Class 1;   *Italic* = Class 2;   Roman = Class 3

Calan. See Verapamil
Calcium channel blockers
Amiodarone 53
Amprenavir 53
Aprepitant 53
Atazanavir 53
Barbiturates 51
Carbamazepine 51
Clarithromycin 52
Conivaptan 53
Cyclosporine 53
Darunavir 53
Delavirdine 53
Diltiazem 53
Efavirenz 51
Erythromycin 52
Fluconazole 52
Fluvoxamine 51
Grapefruit 53
Indinavir 53
Itraconazole 52
Ketoconazole 52
Nafcillin 51
Nefazodone 51
Nelfinavir 53
Nevirapine 51
Oxcarbazepine 51
Phenytoin 51
Posaconazole 52
Primidone 51
Quinupristin 52
Rifabutin 51
Rifampin 51
Rifapentine 51
Ritonavir 53
St. John's Wort 51
Saquinavir 53
Telithromycin 52
Troleandomycin 52
Verapamil 53
Vinblastine 111
Vincristine 111
Vinorelbine 111
Voriconazole 52
Calcium Polycarbophil
Ciprofloxacin 95
Enoxacin 95

Gemifloxacin 95
Levofloxacin 95
Lomefloxacin 95
Moxifloxacin 95
Mycophenolate 85
Norfloxacin 95
Ofloxacin 95
Sparfloxacin 95
Calcium Salts. See Antacids
Candesartan. See Angiotensin
  Receptor Blockers
Capecitabine
Acenocoumarol 31
Chlorpropamide 36
Fosphenytoin 87
Glimepiride 36
Glipizide 36
Glyburide 36
Nateglinide 36
Phenytoin 87
Rosiglitazone 36
Tolbutamide 36
Warfarin 31
Capoten. See ACE Inhibitors
Captopril. See ACE Inhibitors
Carafate. See Sucralfate
Carbamazepine
Acenocoumarol 27
Acetaminophen 21
Alfentanil 81
Amiodarone 24,55
Amlodipine 51
Amprenavir 55,90
Antidepressants,
  tricyclic 32
Aprepitant 55
Aripiprazole 43
Atazanavir 55,90
Atorvastatin 73
Bepridil 51
Cimetidine 55
Clarithromycin 54
Conivaptan 55
Contraceptives, oral 60
Corticosteroids 64
Cyclosporine 55,74
Danazol 55

Darunavir 55,90
Dasatinib 109
Delavirdine 55,90
Diltiazem 51,54
Disopyramide 24
Dronedarone 24
Erlotinib 109
Erythromycin 54
Felodipine 51
Fentanyl 81
Fluconazole 54
Fluoxetine 53
Fluvoxamine 53
Gefitinib 109
Grapefruit 55
Imatinib 109
Indinavir 55,90
Isoniazid 55
Isradipine 51
Itraconazole 47,54
Ketoconazole 47,54
Lamotrigine 76
Lapatinib 109
Lopinavir 90
Lovastatin 73
Methadone 81
Morphine 81
Nefazodone 53
Nelfinavir 55,90
Nicardipine 51
Nifedipine 51
Nilotinib 109
Nimodipine 51
Nisoldipine 51
Nitrendipine 51
Oxycodone 81
Pazopanib 109
Phenprocoumon 27
Posaconazole 47,54
Propoxyphene 55
Quetiapine 92
Quinidine 24
Quinupristin 54
Ritonavir 55,90
Saquinavir 55,90
Simvastatin 73
Sirolimus 74

Underline = Class 1;   *Italic* = Class 2;   Roman = Class 3

Sorafenib 109
Sufentanil 81
Sunitinib 109
Tacrolimus 74
Telithromycin 54
Theophylline 102
Tipranavir 90
Troleandomycin 54
Verapamil 51,54
Voriconazole 47,54
Warfarin 27
Zidovudine 112
Carbenicillin
   Methotrexate 84
Cardene. See Nicardipine
Cardioquin. See Quinidine
Cardizem. See Diltiazem
Carteolol
   Chlorpropamide 34
   Epinephrine 49
   Glimepiride 34
   Glipizide 34
   Glyburide 34
   Insulin 34
   Metformin 34
   Nateglinide 34
   Pioglitazone 34
   Repaglinide 34
   Rosiglitazone 34
   Saxagliptin 34
   Tolbutamide 34
Cartrol. See Carteolol
Carvedilol
   Amiodarone 50
   Bupropion 49
   Chlorpropamide 34
   Cimetidine 50
   Cinacalcet 50
   Diphenhydramine 50
   Duloxetine 49
   Epinephrine 49
   Fluoxetine 49
   Glimepiride 34
   Glipizide 34
   Glyburide 34
   Haloperidol 50
   Insulin 34

Metformin 34
Nateglinide 34
Paroxetine 49
Pioglitazone 34
Propafenone 50
Propoxyphene 50
Quinidine 50
Repaglinide 34
Ritonavir 50
Rosiglitazone 34
Saxagliptin 34
Terbinafine 50
Thioridazine 50
Tolbutamide 34
Catapres. See Clonidine
Cefditoren
   Antacids 56
   Cimetidine 56
   Deslansoprazole 56
   Esomeprazole 56
   Famotidine 56
   Lansoprazole 56
   Nizatidine 56
   Omeprazole 56
   Pantoprazole 56
   Rabeprazole 56
   Ranitidine 56
Cefpodoxime
   Antacids 56
   Cimetidine 56
   Deslansoprazole 56
   Esomeprazole 56
   Famotidine 56
   Lansoprazole 56
   Nizatidine 56
   Omeprazole 56
   Pantoprazole 56
   Rabeprazole 56
   Ranitidine 56
Ceftin. See Cefuroxime
Cefuroxime
   Antacids 56
   Cimetidine 56
   Deslansoprazole 56
   Esomeprazole 56
   Famotidine 56
   Lansoprazole 56

Nizatidine 56
Omeprazole 56
Pantoprazole 56
Rabeprazole 56
Ranitidine 56
Celecoxib
   Lithium 77
Celestone. See
  Betamethasone
Celexa. See Citalopram
CellCept. See Mycophenolate
Centrex. See Prazepam
Cerebyx. See Phenytoin
Chloramphenicol
   Acenocoumarol 30
   Phenytoin 87
   Warfarin 30
Chloromycetin. See
  Chloramphenicol
Chloroquine
   Cyclosporine 75
   Sirolimus 75
   Tacrolimus 75
   Thioridazine 105
Chlorothiazide. See Thiazide
  Diuretics
Chlorpromazine. See
  Phenothiazines and QTc
  table
Chlorpropamide
   Amiodarone 36
   Capecitabine 36
   Carteolol 34
   Carvedilol 34
   Co-trimoxazole 32
   Delavirdine 36
   Efavirenz 36
   Fluconazole 35
   Fluorouracil 36
   Fluoxetine 36
   Fluvastatin 36
   Fluvoxamine 36
   Labetalol 34
   Metronidazole 36
   Nadolol 34
   Penbutolol 34
   Pindolol 34

Underline = Class 1;   *Italic* = Class 2;   Roman = Class 3

Propranolol 34
Sotalol 34
Sulfinpyrazone 36
Timolol 34
Voriconazole 35
Chlorthalidone. See Thiazide
Diuretics
Cholestyramine
Acenocoumarol 27
Bumetanide 65
Furosemide 65
Mycophenolate 85
Phenprocoumon 27
Thiazide Diuretics 65
Thyroid 106
Torsemide 65
Warfarin 27
Cialis. See Tadalafil
Cimetidine
Acenocoumarol 29
Alfentanil 83
Antidepressants,
tricyclic 34
Carbamazepine 55
Carvedilol 50
Cefditoren 56
Cefpodoxime 56
Cefuroxime 56
Clozapine 57
Codeine 58
Dihydrocodeine 58
Dofetilide 66
Fentanyl 83
Glipizide 38
Glyburide 38
Hydrocodone 58
Itraconazole 48
Ketoconazole 48
Methadone 83
Metoprolol 50
Nebivolol 50
Olanzapine 57
Oxycodone 83
Phenytoin 87
Procainamide 89
Propranolol 50
Sildenafil 100

Sufentanil 83
Tadalafil 100
Tamoxifen 101
Theophylline 103
Thioridazine 105
Timolol 50
Tizanidine 106
Vardenafil 100
Warfarin 29
Cinacalcet
Antidepressants,
tricyclic 34
Aripiprazole 46
Carvedilol 50
Codeine 58
Dihydrocodeine 58
Flecainide 25
Hydrocodone 58
Metoprolol 50
Mexiletine 25
Nebivolol 50
Propafenone 25
Propranolol 50
Tamoxifen 101
Thioridazine 105
Timolol 50
Cipro. See Ciprofloxacin
Ciprofloxacin
Antacids 95
Calcium Polycarbophil 95
Clozapine 57
Didanosine 95
Iron 95
Methotrexate 84
Olanzapine 57
Pralatrexate 84
Sucralfate 95
Theophylline 103
Tizanidine 106
Zinc 95
Cisapride. See QTc table
Citalopram
Diclofenac 86
Diflunisal 86
Etodolac 86
Fenoprofen 86
Flurbiprofen 86

<u>Furazolidone</u> 78
Ibuprofen 86
Indomethacin 86
<u>Isocarboxazid</u> 78
Ketoprofen 86
Ketorolac 86
Linezolid 80
Meclofenamate 86
Mefenamic acid 86
Meloxicam 86
Meperidine 83
<u>Methylene Blue</u> 78
Nabumetone 86
Naproxen 86
Oxaprozin 86
<u>Phenelzine</u> 78
Piroxicam 86
Rasagiline 80
Selegiline 80
Sulindac 86
Thiazide Diuretics 10
Tolmetin 86
Tramadol 83
<u>Tranylcypromine</u> 79
Clarithromycin
Alfentanil 82
Alfuzosin 21
Alprazolam 41
Amiodarone 22
Amlodipine 52
Amprenavir 90
Aripiprazole 44
Atazanavir 90
Atorvastatin 71
Bepridil 52
Budesonide 62
Buspirone 41
Carbamazepine 54
Clonazepam 41
Clorazepate 41
Colchicine 59
Corticosteroids 62
Cyclosporine 75
Darunavir 90
Dasatinib 108
Delavirdine 90
Dexamethasone 62

<u>Underline</u> = Class 1;   *Italic* = Class 2;   Roman = Class 3

Diazepam 41
Digoxin 65
Diltiazem 52
Disopyramide 22
Dronedarone 22
Eplerenone 67
Ergot Alkaloids 69
Erlotinib 108
Estazolam 41
Felodipine 52
Fentanyl 82
Flurazepam 41
Fluticasone 62
Gefitinib 108
Halazepam 41
Imatinib 108
Indinavir 90
Isradipine 52
Lapatinib 108
Lopinavir 90
Lovastatin 71
Methadone 82
Methylprednisolone 62
Midazolam 41
Nateglinide 36
Nelfinavir 90
Nicardipine 52
Nifedipine 52
Nilotinib 108
Nimodipine 52
Nisoldipine 52
Nitrendipine 52
Oxycodone 82
Pazopanib 108
Pimozide 87
Pioglitazone 36
Prazepam 41
Quetiapine 93
Quinidine 22
Ranolazine 95
Repaglinide 36
Rifabutin 97
Ritonavir 90
Saquinavir 90
Saxagliptin 36
Sildenafil 99
Simvastatin 71

Sirolimus 75
Sorafenib 108
Sufentanil 82
Sunitinib 108
Tacrolimus 75
Tadalafil 99
Theophylline 103
Tipranavir 90
Triazolam 41
Vardenafil 99
Verapamil 52
Vinblastine 110
Vincristine 110
Vinorelbine 110
Clinoril. See Sulindac
Clomipramine. See Also
    Antidepressants, tricyclic
    and QTc table
    Diclofenac 86
    Diflunisal 86
    Etodolac 86
    Fenoprofen 86
    Flurbiprofen 86
    Furazolidone 78
    Ibuprofen 86
    Indomethacin 86
    Isocarboxazid 78
    Ketoprofen 86
    Ketorolac 86
    Linezolid 79
    Meclofenamate 86
    Mefenamic acid 86
    Meloxicam 86
    Meperidine 83
    Methylene Blue 78
    Nabumetone 86
    Naproxen 86
    Oxaprozin 86
    Phenelzine 78
    Piroxicam 86
    Rasagiline 79
    Selegiline 79
    Sulindac 86
    Thiazide Diuretics 104
    Tolmetin 86
    Tramadol 83
    Tranylcypromine 78

Clonazepam
    Amiodarone 43
    Amprenavir 43
    Aprepitant 43
    Atazanavir 43
    Clarithromycin 41
    Conivaptan 43
    Cyclosporine 43
    Darunavir 43
    Delavirdine 43
    Diltiazem 42
    Erythromycin 41
    Fluconazole 41
    Fluvoxamine 40
    Grapefruit 43
    Indinavir 43
    Itraconazole 41
    Ketoconazole 41
    Nefazodone 40
    Nelfinavir 43
    Posaconazole 41
    Quinupristin 41
    Ritonavir 43
    Saquinavir 43
    Telithromycin 41
    Troleandomycin 41
    Verapamil 42
    Voriconazole 41
Clotrimazole
    Alfentanil 82
    Cyclosporine 75
    Fentanyl 82
    Methadone 82
    Oxycodone 82
    Sirolimus 75
    Sufentanil 82
    Tacrolimus 75
Clonidine
    Amitriptyline 56
    Amoxapine 56
    Clomipramine 56
    Desipramine 56
    Doxepin 56
    Imipramine 56
    Mirtazapine 56
    Nortriptyline 56
    Protriptyline 56

Underline = Class 1;   *Italic* = Class 2;   Roman = Class 3

<u>Underline</u> = Class 1;   *Italic* = Class 2;   Roman = Class 3

Eplerenone 68
Ergot Alkaloids 70
Erlotinib 109
Estazolam 43
Felodipine 53
Fentanyl 83
Flurazepam 43
Gefitinib 109
Halazepam 43
Imatinib 109
Indinavir 92
Isradipine 53
Lapatinib 109
Lopinavir 92
Lovastatin 73
Methadone 83
Midazolam 43
Nateglinide 38
Nelfinavir 92
Nicardipine 53
Nifedipine 53
Nilotinib 109
Nimodipine 53
Nisoldipine 53
Nitrendipine 53
Oxycodone 83
Pazopanib 109
Pimozide 88
Pioglitazone 38
Prazepam 43
Quetiapine 94
Quinidine 24
Ranolazine 96
Repaglinide 38
Rifabutin 98
Ritonavir 92
Saquinavir 92
Saxagliptin 38
Sildenafil 100
Simvastatin 73
Sirolimus 75
Sorafenib 109
Sufentanil 83
Sunitinib 109
Tacrolimus 75
Tadalafil 100
Tipranavir 92

Triazolam 43
Vardenafil 100
Verapamil 53
Vinblastine 111
Vincristine 111
Vinorelbine 111
Contraceptives, Oral
Amoxicillin 61
Ampicillin 61
Antibiotics, oral 61
Barbiturates 60
Bexarotene 60
Bosentan 60
Carbamazepine 60
Clozapine 57
Cyclosporine 75
Efavirenz 60
Felbamate 60
Griseofulvin 60
Modafinil 60
Nafcillin 60
Nevirapine 60
Olanzapine 57
Oxcarbazepine 60
Phenytoin 60
Primidone 60
Rifabutin 60
Rifampin 60
Rifapentine 60
Ritonavir 60
St. John's Wort 60
Sirolimus 75
Tacrolimus 75
Tetracyclines 61
Topiramate 60
Cordarone. See Amiodarone
Coreg. See Carvedilol
Corgard. See Nadolol
Cortef. See Corticosteroids
Corticosteroids
Amiodarone 63
Amprenavir 63
Aprepitant 63
Atazanavir 63
Barbiturates 64
Carbamazepine 64
Clarithromycin 62

Conivaptan 63
Cyclosporine 63
Darunavir 63
Delavirdine 63
Diltiazem 63
Efavirenz 64
Erythromycin 62
Fluconazole 62
Fluvoxamine 62
Grapefruit 63
Indinavir 63
Itraconazole 62
Ketoconazole 62
Nefazodone 62
Nelfinavir 63
Nevirapine 64
Oxcarbazepine 64
Phenytoin 64
Posaconazole 62
Primidone 64
Rifabutin 64
Rifampin 64
Rifapentine 64
Ritonavir 63
Ritonavir 62
Saquinavir 63
St. John's Wort 64
Topiramate 64
Telithromycin 62
Troleandomycin 62
Verapamil 63
Voriconazole 62
Cortisone. See
  Corticosteroids
Cortone. See Corticosteroids
Co-trimoxazole
Acenocoumarol 30
Chlorpropamide 36
Glimepiride 36
Glipizide 36
Glyburide 36
Methotrexate 84
Nateglinide 36
Pralatrexate 84
Phenytoin 87
Procainamide 89
Rosiglitazone 36

Underline = Class 1;   *Italic* = Class 2;   Roman = Class 3

<u>Underline</u> = Class 1;   *Italic* = Class 2;   Roman = Class 3

Danshen. See Herbal
Interaction chart

Darunavir
Alfentanil 83
Alfuzosin 22
Alprazolam 43
Amiodarone 24,92
Amlodipine 53
Amprenavir 92
Aprepitant 92
Aripiprazole 45
Atazanavir 92
Atorvastatin 73
Barbiturates 84
Bepridil 53
Bosentan 90
Buspirone 43
Carbamazepine 55,90
Clarithromycin 90
Clonazepam 43
Clorazepate 43
Conivaptan 92
Corticosteroids 63
Cyclosporine 75,92
Dasatinib 109
Delavirdine 92
Diazepam 43
Diltiazem 53,92
Disopyramide 24
Dronedarone 24
Efavirenz 90
Eplerenone 68
Ergot Alkaloids 70
Erlotinib 109
Erythromycin 90
Estazolam 43
Felodipine 53
Fentanyl 83
Fluconazole 90
Flurazepam 43
Fluvoxamine 91
Gefitinib 109
Grapefruit 92
Halazepam 43
Imatinib 109
Indinavir 92
Isradipine 53

Itraconazole 90
Ketoconazole 90
Lapatinib 109
Lopinavir 92
Lovastatin 73
Methadone 83
Midazolam 43
Nateglinide 38
Nefazodone 91
Nelfinavir 92
Nevirapine 90
Nicardipine 53
Nifedipine 53
Nilotinib 109
Nimodipine 53
Nisoldipine 53
Nitrendipine 53
Oxcarbazepine 90
Oxycodone 83
Pazopanib 109
Phenytoin 90
Pimozide 88
Pioglitazone 38
Posaconazole 90
Prazepam 43
Primidone 90
Quetiapine 94
Quinidine 24
Quinupristin 90
Ranolazine 96
Repaglinide 38
Rifabutin 90,98
Rifampin 90
Rifapentine 90
Ritonavir 92
Saquinavir 92
Saxagliptin 38
Sildenafil 100
Simvastatin 73
Sirolimus 75
Sorafenib 109
St. John's Wort 90
Sufentanil 83
Sunitinib 109
Tacrolimus 75
Tadalafil 100
Telithromycin 90

Tipranavir 92
Triazolam 43
Troleandomycin 90
Vardenafil 100
Verapamil 53,92
Vinblastine 111
Vincristine 111
Vinorelbine 111
Voriconazole 90
Darvon. See Propoxyphene

Dasatinib
Amiodarone 109
Amprenavir 109
Aprepitant 109
Atazanavir 109
Barbiturates 109
Carbamazepine 109
Clarithromycin 108
Conivaptan 109
Cyclosporine 109
Darunavir 109
Delavirdine 109
Diltiazem 109
Efavirenz 109
Erythromycin
Fluconazole 108
Fluvoxamine 107
Grapefruit 109
Indinavir 109
Isoniazid 108
Itraconazole 108
Ketoconazole 108
Nefazodone 107
Nelfinavir 109
Nevirapine 109
Oxcarbazepine 109
Phenytoin 109
Posaconazole 108
Primidone 109
Quinupristin 108
Rifabutin 109
Rifampin 109
Rifapentine109
Ritonavir 109
Saquinavir 109
St. John's Wort 109
Telithromycin 108

Underline = Class 1;   *Italic* = Class 2;   Roman = Class 3

Underline = Class 1;   *Italic* = Class 2;   Roman = Class 3

Azithromycin 65
Bepridil 64
Clarithromycin 65
Conivaptan 65
Cyclosporine 65
Diltiazem 64
Erythromycin 65
Hydroxychloroquine 65
Indinavir 65
Itraconazole 65
Ketoconazole 65
Nelfinavir 65
Posaconazole 65
Propafenone 65
Quinidine 65
Ranolazine 65
Ritonavir 65
Saquinavir 65
Tacrolimus 65
Tamoxifen 65
Telithromycin 65
Verapamil 64
Dihydrocodeine
Amiodarone 58
Bupropion 58
Cimetidine 58
Cinacalcet 58
Diphenhydramine 58
Duloxetine 58
Fluoxetine 58
Haloperidol 58
Paroxetine 58
Propafenone 58
Propoxyphene 58
Quinidine 58
Ritonavir 58
Terbinafine 58
Thioridazine 58
Dihydroergotamine. See
Ergot Alkaloids
Dilantin. See Phenytoin
Diltiazem. See also Calcium
channel blockers
Alfentanil 83
Alfuzosin 22
Alprazolam 42
Amiodarone 23

Amlodipine 53
Amprenavir 92
Aripiprazole 45
Atazanavir 92
Atorvastatin 71
Bepridil 53
Buspirone 42
Carbamazepine 51,54
Clonazepam 42
Clorazepate 42
Colchicine 60
Corticosteroids 63
Cyclosporine 75
Darunavir 92
Dasatinib 109
Delavirdine 92
Diazepam 42
Digoxin 64
Disopyramide 23
Dronedarone 23
Eplerenone 68
Ergot Alkaloids 70
Erlotinib 109
Estazolam 42
Felodipine 53
Fentanyl 83
Flurazepam 42
Gefitinib 109
Halazepam 42
Imatinib 109
Indinavir 92
Isradipine 53
Lapatinib 109
Lopinavir 92
Lovastatin 71
Methadone 83
Midazolam 42
Nateglinide 37
Nelfinavir 92
Nicardipine 53
Nifedipine 53
Nilotinib 109
Nimodipine 53
Nisoldipine 53
Nitrendipine 53
Oxycodone 83
Pazopanib 109

<u>Pimozide</u> 88
Pioglitazone 37
Prazepam 42
Quetiapine 94
Quinidine 23
Ranolazine 96
Repaglinide 37
Rifabutin 51,98
Ritonavir 92
Saquinavir 92
Saxagliptin 37
Sildenafil 99
Simvastatin 71
Sirolimus 75
Sorafenib 109
Sufentanil 83
Sunitinib 109
Tacrolimus 75
Tadalafil 99
Tipranavir 92
Triazolam 42
Vardenafil 99
Verapamil 53
Vinblastine 111
Vincristine 111
Vinorelbine 111
Diovan. See Angiotensin
Receptor Blockers
Diphenhydramine
Antidepressants,
tricyclic 34
Aripiprazole 46
Carvedilol 50
Codeine 58
Dihydrocodeine 58
Flecainide 25
Hydrocodone 58
Metoprolol 50
Mexiletine 25
Nebivolol 50
Propafenone 25
Propranolol 50
Tamoxifen 101
Thioridazine 105
Timolol 50
Disopyramide. See also
table

<u>Underline</u> = Class 1;   *Italic* = Class 2;   Roman = Class 3

<u>Underline</u> = Class 1;   *Italic* = Class 2;   Roman = Class 3

Underline = Class 1;   *Italic* = Class 2;   Roman = Class 3

<u>Underline</u> = Class 1;   *Italic* = Class 2;   Roman = Class 3

Felodipine 52
Fentanyl 82
Flurazepam 41
Fluticasone 62
Gefitinib 108
Halazepam 41
Imatinib 108
Indinavir 90
Isradipine 52
Lapatinib 108
Lopinavir 90
Lovastatin 71
Methadone 82
Methylprednisolone 62
Midazolam 41
Nateglinide 36
Nelfinavir 90
Nicardipine 52
Nifedipine 52
Nilotinib 108
Nimodipine 52
Nisoldipine 52
Nitrendipine 52
Oxycodone 82
Pazopanib 108
<u>Pimozide</u> 87
Pioglitazone 36
Prazepam 41
Quetiapine 93
Quinidine 22
Ranolazine 95
Repaglinide 36
Rifabutin 97
Ritonavir 90
Saquinavir 90
Saxagliptin 36
Sildenafil 99
Simvastatin 71
Sirolimus 75
Sorafenib 108
Sufentanil 82
Sunitinib 108
Tacrolimus 75
Tadalafil 99
Theophylline 103
Tipranavir 90
Triazolam 41

Vardenafil 99
Verapamil 52
Vinblastine 110
Vincristine 110
Vinorelbine 110
Escitalopram
  Diclofenac 86
  Diflunisal 86
  Etodolac 86
  Fenoprofen 86
  Flurbiprofen 86
  Fluvoxamine 40
  <u>Furazolidone</u> 78
  Ibuprofen 86
  Indomethacin 86
  <u>Isocarboxazid</u> 78
  Ketoprofen 86
  Ketorolac 86
  Linezolid 80
  Meclofenamate 86
  Mefenamic acid 86
  Meloxicam 86
  Meperidine 83
  <u>Methylene Blue</u> 78
  Nabumetone 86
  Naproxen 86
  Oxaprozin 86
  <u>Phenelzine</u> 78
  Piroxicam 86
  Rasagiline 80
  Selegiline 80
  Sulindac 86
  Thiazide Diuretics 104
  Tolmetin 86
  Tramadol 83
  <u>Tranylcypromine</u> 78
Eskalith. See Lithium
Esomeprazole
  Cefditoren 56
  Cefpodoxime 56
  Cefuroxime 56
  Glipizide 38
  Glyburide 38
  Itraconazole 48
  Ketoconazole 48
Estazolam
  Amiodarone 43

Amprenavir 43
Aprepitant 43
Atazanavir 43
Clarithromycin 41
Conivaptan 43
Cyclosporine 43
Darunavir 43
Delavirdine 43
Diltiazem 42
Erythromycin 41
Fluconazole 41
Fluvoxamine 40
Grapefruit 43
Indinavir 43
Itraconazole 41
Ketoconazole 41
Nefazodone 40
Nelfinavir 43
Quinupristin 41
Ritonavir 43
Saquinavir 43
Telithromycin 41
Troleandomycin 41
Verapamil 42
Voriconazole 41
Ethacrynic Acid
  Lithium 77
Ethanol. See Alcohol
Etodolac
  Acenocoumarol 31
  ACE Inhibitors 39
  Angiotensin Receptor
    Blockers 39
  Citalopram 86
  Clomipramine 86
  Duloxetine 86
  Escitalopram 86
  Fluoxetine 86
  Fluvoxamine 86
  Lithium 77
  Methotrexate 84
  Milnacipran 86
  Nefazodone 86
  Paroxetine 86
  Phenprocoumon 31
  Pralatrexate 84
  Sertraline 86

<u>Underline</u> = Class 1;   *Italic* = Class 2;   Roman = Class 3

Venlafaxine 86
Warfarin 31
Etrafon. See Phenothiazines
Etravirine
  Atorvastatin 73
  Lovastatin 73
  Simvastatin 73
Exna. See Benzthiazide
Factive. See Gemifloxacin
Febuxostat
  <u>Azathioprine</u> 40
  <u>Mercaptopurine</u> 40
  Theophylline 103
Famotidine
  Cefditoren 56
  Cefpodoxime 56
  Cefuroxime 56
  Glipizide 38
  Glyburide 38
  Itraconazole 48
  Ketoconazole 48
Felbamate
  Contraceptives, oral 60
Felbatol. See Felbamate
Feldene. See Piroxicam
Felodipine. See Calcium
  channel blockers
Fenofibrate
  Acenocoumarol 31
  Warfarin 31
Fenoprofen
  Acenocoumarol 31
  ACE Inhibitors 39
  Angiotensin Receptor
    Blockers 39
  Citalopram 86
  Clomipramine 86
  Duloxetine 86
  Escitalopram 86
  Fluoxetine 86
  Fluvoxamine 86
  Lithium 77
  Methotrexate 84
  Milnacipran 86
  Nefazodone 86
  Paroxetine 86
  Phenprocoumon 31

Pralatrexate 84
Sertraline 86
Venlafaxine 86
Warfarin 31
Fentanyl
  Amiodarone 83
  Amprenavir 83
  Atazanavir 83
  Barbiturates 81
  Bosentan 81
  Carbamazepine 81
  Cimetidine 83
  Citalopram 83
  Clarithromycin 82
  Clomipramine 83
  Clotrimazole 82
  Conivaptan 83
  Cyclosporine 83
  Darunavir 83
  Delavirdine 83
  Desvenlafaxine 83
  Diltiazem 83
  Duloxetine 83
  Efavirenz 81
  Erythromycin 82
  Escitalopram 83
  Fluconazole 82
  Fluoxetine 83
  Fluvoxamine 83
  Fluvoxamine 83
  <u>Furazolidone</u> 78
  Grapefruit 83
  Imipramine 83
  Indinavir 83
  <u>Isocarboxazid</u> 78
  Itraconazole 82
  Ketoconazole 82
  Linezolid 80
  <u>Methylene Blue</u> 78
  Milnacipran 83
  Nefazodone 83
  Nelfinavir 83
  Nevirapine 81
  Oxcarbamazepine 81
  Paroxetine 83
  <u>Phenelzine</u> 78
  Phenytoin 81

Posaconazole 82
Primidone 81
Quinupristin 82
Rasagiline 80
Rifampin 81
Rifapentine 81
Ritonavir 81,83
Saquinavir 83
Selegiline 80
Sertraline 81
St. John's Wort 81
Telithromycin 82
<u>Tranylcypromine</u> 78
Troleandomycin 82
Venlafaxine 83
Verapamil 83
Voriconazole 82
Ferrous Sulfate. See Iron
Ferrous Gluconate. See Iron
Feverfew. See Herbal
  Interaction chart
Flagyl. See Metronidazole
Flecainide
  Amiodarone 25
  Bupropion 25
  Cinacalcet 25
  Diphenhydramine 25
  Duloxetine 25
  Fluoxetine 25
  Haloperidol 25
  Paroxetine 25
  Propafenone 25
  Propoxyphene 25
  Quinidine 25
  Ritonavir 25
  Terbinafine 25
  Thioridazine 25
Flexeril. See
  Cyclobenzaprine
Flovent. See Corticosteroids
Floxin. See Ofloxacin
Fluconazole
  Acenocoumarol 27
  Alfentanil 82
  Alfuzosin 21
  Alprazolam 41
  Amiodarone 22

<u>Underline</u> = Class 1;   *Italic* = Class 2;   Roman = Class 3

Amlodipine 52
Amprenavir 90
Aripiprazole 44
Atazanavir 90
Atorvastatin 71
Bepridil 52
Budesonide 62
Buspirone 41
Carbamazepine 54
Chlorpropamide 35
Clonazepam 41
Clorazepate 41
Colchicine 59
Corticosteroids 62
Cyclosporine 75
Darunavir 90
Dasatinib 108
Delavirdine 90
Dexamethasone 62
Diazepam 41
Diltiazem 52
Disopyramide 22
Dronedarone 22
Eplerenone 67
Ergot Alkaloids 69
Erlotinib 108
Estazolam 41
Felodipine 52
Fentanyl 82
Flurazepam 41
Fluticasone 62
Gefitinib 108
Glimepiride 35
Glipizide 35
Glyburide 35
Halazepam 41
Imatinib 108
Indinavir 90
Isradipine 52
Lapatinib 108
Lopinavir 90
Lovastatin 71
Methadone 82
Methylprednisolone 62
Midazolam 41
Nateglinide 35
Nelfinavir 90

Nicardipine 52
Nifedipine 52
Nilotinib 108
Nimodipine 52
Nisoldipine 52
Nitrendipine 52
Oxycodone 82
Pazopanib 108
Phenytoin 87
<u>Pimozide</u> 87
Pioglitazone 36
Prazepam 41
Quetiapine 93
Quinidine 22
Ranolazine 95
Repaglinide 36
Rifabutin 97
Ritonavir 90
Rosiglitazone 35
Saquinavir 90
Saxagliptin 36
Sildenafil 99
Simvastatin 71
Sirolimus 75
Sorafenib 108
Sufentanil 82
Sunitinib 108
Tacrolimus 75
Tadalafil 99
Tipranavir 90
Tolbutamide 35
Triazolam 41
Vardenafil 99
Verapamil 52
Vinblastine 110
Vincristine 110
Vinorelbine 110
Warfarin 27

Fluorouracil
Acenocoumarol 31
Chlorpropamide 36
Fosphenytoin 87
Glimepiride 36
Glipizide 36
Glyburide 36
Nateglinide 36
Phenytoin 87

Rosiglitazone 36
Tolbutamide 36
Warfarin 31

Fluoxetine
Acenocoumarol 30
Antidepressants,
tricyclic 33
Aripiprazole 45
Carbamazepine 53
Carvedilol 49
Chlorpropamide 36
Codeine 58
Diclofenac 86
Diflunisal 86
Dihydrocodeine 58
Etodolac 86
Fenoprofen 86
Flecainide 25
Flurbiprofen 86
<u>Furazolidone</u> 78
Glimepiride 36
Glipizide 36
Glyburide 36
Hydrocodone 58
Ibuprofen 86
Indomethacin 86
<u>Isocarboxazid</u> 78
Ketoprofen 86
Ketorolac 86
Linezolid 80
Meclofenamate 86
Mefenamic acid 86
Meloxicam 86
Meperidine 83
<u>Methylene Blue</u> 78
Metoprolol 49
Mexiletine 25
Nabumetone 86
Naproxen 86
Nateglinide 36
Nebivolol 49
<u>Phenelzine</u> 78
Phenytoin 87
Piroxicam 86
Propafenone 25
Propranolol 49
Rasagiline 80

<u>Underline</u> = Class 1;   *Italic* = Class 2;   Roman = Class 3

Nabumetone 86
Naproxen 86
Nateglinide 36,38
Nelfinavir 91
Nicardipine 51
Nifedipine 51
Nilotinib 107
Nimodipine 51
Nisoldipine 51
Nitrendipine 51
Olanzapine 57
Oxaprozin 86
Oxycodone 83
Pazopanib 107
<u>Phenelzine</u> 78
Phenytoin 87
<u>Pimozide</u> 88
Pioglitazone 38
Piroxicam 86
Prazepam 40
Quetiapine 94
Quinidine 23
Ranolazine 96
Rasagiline 80
Repaglinide 38
Rifabutin 97
Ritonavir 91
Rosiglitazone 36
Saquinavir 91
Saxagliptin 38
Selegiline 80
Sildenafil 98
Simvastatin 73
Sirolimus 75
Sorafenib 107
Sufentanil 83
Sulindac 86
Sunitinib 107
Tacrolimus 75
Tadalafil 98
Theophylline 102
Thiazide Diuretics 104
Thioridazine 105
Tipranavir 91
Tizanidine 106
Tolbutamide 36
Tolmetin 86

Tramadol 83
<u>Tranylcypromine</u> 78
Triazolam 40
Vardenafil 98
Verapamil 51
Vinblastine 111
Vincristine 111
Vinorelbine 111
Warfarin 30
Fosamprenavir. See
  Amprenavir
Fosinopril. See ACE
  Inhibitors
Fosphenytoin. See Phenytoin
Frova. See Frovatriptan
Frovatriptan
  <u>Ergot Alkaloids</u> 70
Fulvicin. See Griseofulvin
Furazolidone. See MAO
  Inhibitors
Furoxone. See MAO
  Inhibitors
Furosemide
  Cholestyramine 65
  Colestipol 65
  Lithium 77
Garlic. See Herbal
  Interaction chart
Gaviscon. See Antacids
Gefitinib
  Amiodarone 109
  Amprenavir 109
  Aprepitant 109
  Atazanavir 109
  Barbiturates 109
  Carbamazepine 109
  Clarithromycin 108
  Conivaptan 109
  Cyclosporine 109
  Darunavir 109
  Delavirdine 109
  Diltiazem 109
  Efavirenz 109
  Erythromycin 108
  Fluconazole 108
  Fluvoxamine 107
  Grapefruit 109

Indinavir 109
Isoniazid 108
Itraconazole 108
Ketoconazole 108
Nefazodone 107
Nelfinavir 109
Nevirapine 109
Oxcarbazepine 109
Phenytoin 109
Posaconazole 108
Primidone 109
Quinupristin 108
Rifabutin 109
Rifampin 109
Rifapentine 109
Ritonavir 109
Saquinavir 109
St. John's Wort 109
Telithromycin 108
Troleandomycin 108
Verapamil 109
Voriconazole 108
Gelusil. See Antacids
Gemfibrozil
  Acenocoumarol 31
  Atorvastatin 72
  Lovastatin 72
  Rosuvastatin 72
  Simvastatin 72
  Warfarin 31
Gemifloxacin
  Antacids 95
  Calcium Polycarboph
  Didanosine 95
  Iron 95
  Sucralfate 95
  Zinc 95
Ginger. See Herbal
  Interaction chart
Ginkgo. See Herbal
  Interaction chart
Ginseng. See Herbal
  Interaction chart
Gleevec. See Imatinib
Glimepiride
  Amiodarone 36
  Capecitabine 36

<u>Underline</u> = Class 1;   *Italic* = Class 2;   Roman = Class 3

Carteolol 34
Carvedilol 34
Co-trimoxazole 36
Delavirdine 36
Efavirenz 36
Fluconazole 35
Fluoxetine 36
Fluorouracil 36
Fluvastatin 36
Fluvoxamine 36
Labetalol 34
Metronidazole 36
Nadolol 34
Penbutolol 34
Pindolol 34
Propranolol 34
Timolol 34
Sotalol 34
Sulfinpyrazone 36
Voriconazole 35
Glipizide
Amiodarone 36
Capecitabine 36
Antacids 38
Carteolol 34
Carvedilol 34
Cimetidine 38
Co-trimoxazole 36
Delavirdine 36
Deslansoprazole 38
Efavirenz 36
Esomeprazole 38
Famotidine 38
Fluconazole 35
Fluoxetine 36
Fluorouracil 36
Fluvastatin 36
Fluvoxamine 36
Labetalol 34
Lansoprazole 38
Metronidazole 36
Nadolol 34
Nizatidine 38
Omeprazole 38
Pantoprazole 38
Penbutolol 34
Pindolol 34

Propranolol 34
Rabeprazole 38
Ranitidine 38
Sotalol 34
Sulfinpyrazone 36
Timolol 34
Voriconazole 35
Glucophage. See Metformin
Glucosamine.. See Herbal
   Interaction chart
Glucotrol. See Glipizide
Glucovance. See Glyburide
   and Metformin
Glyburide
Amiodarone 36
Antacids 38
Capecitabine 36
Carteolol 34
Carvedilol 34
Cimetidine 38
Delavirdine 36
Deslansoprazole 38
Efavirenz 36
Esomeprazole 38
Famotidine 38
Fluconazole 35
Fluoxetine 36
Fluorouracil 36
Fluvastatin 36
Fluvoxamine 36
Labetalol 34
Lansoprazole 38
Metronidazole 36
Nadolol 34
Nizatidine 38
Omeprazole 38
Pantoprazole 38
Penbutolol 34
Pindolol 34
Propranolol 34
Rabeprazole 38
Ranitidine 38
Sotalol 34
Sulfinpyrazone 36
Timolol 34
Voriconazole 35
Grapefruit

Alfentanil 83
Alfuzosin 22
Alprazolam 43
Amiodarone 24
Amlodipine 53
Amprenavir 92
Aripiprazole 45
Atorvastatin 73
Atazanavir 92
Bepridil 53
Buspirone 43
Carbamazepine 55
Colchicine 60
Clonazepam 43
Clorazepate 43
Corticosteroids 63
Cyclosporine 75
Darunavir 92
Dasatinib 109
Delavirdine 92
Diazepam 43
Diltiazem 53
Disopyramide 24
Dronedarone 24
Eplerenone 68
Ergot Alkaloids 70
Erlotinib 109
Estazolam 43
Felodipine 53
Fentanyl 83
Flurazepam 43
Gefitinib 109
Halazepam 43
Imatinib 109
Indinavir 92
Isradipine 53
Lapatinib 109
Lovastatin 73
Methadone 83
Midazolam 43
Nateglinide 38
Nelfinavir 92
Nicardipine 53
Nifedipine 53
Nilotinib 109
Nimodipine 53
Nisoldipine 53

<u>Underline</u> = Class 1;   *Italic* = Class 2;   Roman = Class 3

Nitrendipine 53
Oxycodone 83
Pazopanib 109
<u>Pimozide</u> 88
Pioglitazone 38
Prazepam 43
Quetiapine 94
Quinidine 24
Ranolazine 96
Repaglinide 38
Rifabutin 98
Ritonavir 92
Saquinavir 92
Saxagliptin 38
Sildenafil 100
Simvastatin 73
Sirolimus 75
Sorafenib 109
Sufentanil 83
Sunitinib 109
Tacrolimus 75
Tadalafil 100
Tipranavir 92
Triazolam 43
Vardenafil 100
Verapamil 53
Vinblastine 111
Vincristine 111
Vinorelbine 111
Green Tea. See Herbal
Interaction chart
Griseofulvin
  Acenocoumarol 27
  Contraceptives, oral 60
  Phenprocoumon 27
  Theophylline 102
  Warfarin 27
Guanabenz
  Amitriptyline 56
  Amoxapine 56
  Clomipramine 56
  Desipramine 56
  Doxepin 56
  Imipramine 56
  Mirtazapine 56
  Nortriptyline 56
  Protriptyline 56

Trimipramine 56
Guanfacine
  Amitriptyline 56
  Amoxapine 56
  Clomipramine 56
  Desipramine 56
  Doxepin 56
  Imipramine 56
  Mirtazaline 56
  Nortriptyline 56
  Protriptyline 56
  Trimipramine 56
Halazepam
  Amiodarone 43
  Amprenavir 43
  Aprepitant 43
  Atazanavir 43
  Clarithromycin 41
  Conivaptan 43
  Cyclosporine 43
  Darunavir 43
  Delavirdine 43
  Diltiazem 42
  Erythromycin 41
  Fluconazole 41
  Fluvoxamine 40
  Grapefruit 43
  Indinavir 43
  Itraconazole 41
  Ketoconazole 41
  Nefazodone 40
  Nelfinavir 43
  Posaconazole 41
  Quinupristin 41
  Ritonavir 43
  Saquinavir 43
  Telithromycin 41
  Troleandomycin 41
  Verapamil 42
  Voriconazole 41
Halcion. See Triazolam
Haldol. See Haloperidol
Haloperidol. See also QTc
table
  Antidepressants,
    tricyclic 34
  Aripiprazole 46

Bromocriptine 66
Cabergoline 66
Carvedilol 50
Codeine 58
Dihydrocodeine 58
Flecainide 25
Hydrocodone 58
Levodopa 66
Metoprolol 50
Mexiletine 25
Nebivolol 50
Pramipexole 66
Propafenone 25
Propranolol 50
Ropinirole 66
Tamoxifen 101
Thioridazine 105
Timolol 50
Hydrochlorothiazide. See
  Thiazide Diuretics
Hydrocodone
  Amiodarone 58
  Bupropion 58
  Cimetidine 58
  Cinacalcet 58
  Diphenhydramine 58
  Duloxetine 58
  Fluoxetine 58
  Haloperidol 58
  Paroxetine 58
  Propafenone 58
  Propoxyphene 58
  Quinidine 58
  Ritonavir 58
  Terbinafine 58
  Thioridazine 58
Hydrocortisone. See
  Corticosteroids
Hydroflumethiazide. See
  Thiazide Diuretics
Hydromox. See
  Quinethazone
Hydroxychloroquine
  Digoxin 65
Hygroton. See Thiazide
  Diuretics
Ibuprofen

<u>Underline</u> = Class 1;   *Italic* = Class 2;   Roman = Class 3

<u>Underline</u> = Class 1; *Italic* = Class 2; Roman = Class 3

Ergot Alkaloids 70
Erlotinib 109
Erythromycin 90
Estazolam 43
Felodipine 53
Fentanyl 83
Fluconazole 90
Flurazepam 43
Fluvoxamine 91
Gefitinib 109
Grapefruit 92
Halazepam 43
Imatinib 109
Isradipine 53
Itraconazole 90
Ketoconazole 90
Lapatinib 109
Lopinavir 92
Lovastatin 73
Methadone 83
Midazolam 43
Nateglinide 38
Nefazodone 91
Nelfinavir 92
Nevirapine 92
Nicardipine 53
Nifedipine 53
Nilotinib 109
Nimodipine 53
Nisoldipine 53
Nitrendipine 53
Oxcarbazepine 90
Oxycodone 83
Pazopanib 109
Phenytoin 90
Pimozide 88
Pioglitazone 38
Posaconazole 90
Prazepam 43
Primidone 90
Quetiapine 94
Quinidine 24
Quinupristin 90
Ranolazine 96
Repaglinide 38
Rifabutin 90,98
Rifampin 90

Rifapentine 90
Ritonavir 92
Saquinavir 92
Saxagliptin 38
Sildenafil 100
Simvastatin 73
Sirolimus 75
Sorafenib 109
St. John's Wort 90
Sufentanil 83
Sunitinib 109
Tacrolimus 75
Tadalafil 100
Telithromycin 90
Tipranavir 92
Triazolam 43
Troleandomycin 90
Vardenafil 100
Verapamil 53,92
Vinblastine 111
Vincristine 111
Vinorelbine 111
Voriconazole 90
Indocin. See Indomethacin
Indomethacin
  Acenocoumarol 31
  ACE Inhibitors 39
  Angiotensin Receptor
   Blockers 39
  Citalopram 86
  Clomipramine 86
  Duloxetine 86
  Escitalopram 86
  Fluoxetine 86
  Fluvoxamine 86
  Lithium 77
  Methotrexate 84
  Milnacipran 86
  Nefazodone 86
  Paroxetine 86
  Phenprocoumon 31
  Pralatrexate 84
  Sertraline 86
  Venlafaxine 86
  Warfarin 31
INH. See Isoniazid
Inspra. See Eplerenone

Insulin
  Carteolol 34
  Carvedilol 34
  Labetalol 34
  Nadolol 34
  Penbutolol 34
  Pindolol 34
  Propranolol 34
  Sotalol 34
  Timolol 34
Intelence. See Etravirine
Invirase. See Saquinavir
Ionamin. See Phentermine
Irbesartan. See Angiotensin
  Receptor Blockers
Iressa. See Gefitinib
Iron
  Ciprofloxacin 95
  Enoxacin 95
  Gemifloxacin 95
  Levofloxacin 95
  Moxifloxacin 95
  Norfloxacin 95
  Sparfloxacin 95
  Tetracyclines 101
  Thyroid 106
Isocarboxazid. See MAO
  Inhibitors, Nonselective
Isometheptene
  <u>Furazolidone</u> 79
  <u>Isocarboxazid</u> 79
  <u>Linezolid</u> 81
  <u>Methylene Blue</u> 79
  <u>Phenelzine</u> 79
  Rasagiline 81
  Selegiline 81
  <u>Tranylcypromine</u> 79
Ismo. See Nitrates
Isoniazid
  Acenocoumarol 31
  Acetaminophen 21
  Carbamazepine 55
  Dasatinib 108
  Erlotinib 108
  Gefitinib 108
  Imatinib 108
  Lapatinib 108

<u>Underline</u> = Class 1; *Italic* = Class 2; Roman = Class 3

<u>Underline</u> = Class 1;   *Italic* = Class 2;   Roman = Class 3

<u>Underline</u> = Class 1; *Italic* = Class 2; Roman = Class 3

Phenylephrine 81
Propoxyphene 80
Pseudoephedrine 81
Sertraline 80
Sibutramine 80
Tapentadol 81
Tetrabenzine 80
Tramadol 80
Trazodone 80
Venlafaxine 80
Liothyronine. See Thyroid
Liotrix. See Thyroid
Lipitor. See Atorvastatin
Lisinopril. See ACE
  Inhibitors
Lithium
  ACE Inhibitors 77
  Angiotensin Receptor
    Blockers 77
  Benazepril 77
  Bumetanide 77
  Captopril 77
  Celecoxib 77
  Diclofenac 77
  Diflunisal 77
  Enalapril 77
  Ethacrynic acid 77
  Etodolac 77
  Fenoprofen 77
  Fosinopril 77
  Furosemide 77
  Ibuprofen 77
  Indomethacin 77
  Ketoprofen 77
  Ketorolac 77
  Lisinopril 77
  Meclofenamate 77
  Mefenamic acid 77
  Moexipril 77
  Nabumetone 77
  Naproxen 77
  Perindopril 77
  Quinapril 77
  Ramipril 77
  Thiazide Diuretics 77
  Tolmetin 77
  Torsemide 77

Trandolapril 77
Valdecoxib 77
Iodine. See Etodolac
Lomefloxacin
  Antacids 95
  Calcium Polycarbophil 95
  Didanosine 95
  Sucralfate 95
  Zinc 95
Lopid. See Gemfibrozil
Lopinavir
  Amprenavir 92
  Amiodarone 92
  Aprepitant 92
  Atazanavir 92
  Barbiturates 90
  Bosentan 90
  Carbamazepine 90
  Clarithromycin 90
  Conivaptan 92
  Cyclosporine 92
  Darunavir 92
  Delavirdine 92
  Diltiazem 92
  Efavirenz 90
  Erythromycin 90
  Fluconazole 90
  Fluvoxamine 91
  Grapefruit 92
  Indinavir 92
  Itraconazole 90
  Ketoconazole 90
  Nefazodone 91
  Nelfinavir 92
  Nevirapine 90
  Oxcarbazepine 90
  Phenytoin 90
  Posaconazole 90
  Primidone 90
  Quinupristin 90
  Rifabutin 90
  Rifampin 90
  Rifapentine 90
  Ritonavir 92
  Saquinavir 92
  St. John's Wort 90
  Telithromycin 90

Troleandomycin 90
Verapamil 92
Voriconazole 90
Lortab. See Hydrocodone
Losartan. See Angiotensin
  Receptor Blockers
Lotensin. See ACE Inhibi
Lovastatin
  Acenocoumarol 28
  Amiodarone 73
  Amprenavir 73
  Atazanavir 73
  Barbiturates 73
  Carbamazepine 73
  Clarithromycin 71
  Conivaptan 73
  Cyclosporine 73
  Darunavir 73
  Delavirdine 73
  Diltiazem 71
  Efavirenz 73
  Erythromycin 71
  Etravirine 73
  Fluvoxamine 73
  Gemfibrozil 72
  Fluconazole 71
  Fluvoxamine 73
  Grapefruit 73
  Imatinib 73
  Indinavir 73
  Itraconazole 71
  Ketoconazole 71
  Nefazodone 73
  Nelfinavir 73
  Nevirapine 73
  Oxcarbazepine 73
  Phenytoin 73
  Posaconazole 71
  Primidone 73
  Quinupristin 71
  Rifabutin 73
  Rifampin 73
  Rifapentine 73
  Ritonavir 73
  St. John's Wort 73
  Saquinavir 73
  Telithromycin 71

<u>Underline</u> = Class 1;   *Italic* = Class 2;   Roman = Class 3

160

Underline = Class 1;   *Italic* = Class 2;   Roman = Class 3

Fluvoxamine 86
Lithium 77
Methotrexate 84
Milnacipran 86
Nefazodone 86
Paroxetine 86
Phenprocoumon 31
Pralatrexate 84
Sertraline 86
Venlafaxine 86
Warfarin 31
Melatonin. See Herbal
Interaction chart
Mefloquine. See QTc table
Acenocoumarol 31
Warfarin 31
Mellaril. See Thioridazine
Meloxicam
Acenocoumarol 31
ACE Inhibitors 39
Angiotensin Receptor
  Blockers 39
Citalopram 86
Clomipramine 86
Duloxetine 86
Escitalopram 86
Fluoxetine 86
Fluvoxamine 86
Lithium 77
Methotrexate 84
Milnacipran 86
Nefazodone 86
Paroxetine 86
Phenprocoumon 31
Pralatrexate 84
Sertraline 86
Venlafaxine 86
Warfarin 31
Meperidine
Citalopram 83
Clomipramine 83
Desvenlafaxine 83
Duloxetine 83
Escitalopram 83
<u>Furazolidone</u> 78
Fluoxetine 83
Fluvoxamine 83

Imipramine 83
<u>Isocarboxazid</u> 78
Linezolid 80
<u>Methylene Blue</u> 78
Milnacipran 83
Paroxetine 83
<u>Phenelzine</u> 78
Rasagiline 80
Selegiline 80
Sertraline 83
<u>Tranylcypromine</u> 78
Venlafaxine 83
Mercaptopurine
<u>Allopurinol</u> 40
<u>Febuxostat</u> 40
Meridia. See Sibutramine
Meropenem
<u>Valproic Acid</u> 110
Merrem. See Meropenem
Mesoridazine. See QTc table
Metaraminol
<u>Furazolidone</u> 79
<u>Isocarboxazid</u> 79
Linezolid 81
<u>Methylene Blue</u> 79
<u>Phenelzine</u> 79
Rasagiline 81
Selegiline 81
<u>Tranylcypromine</u> 79
Metformin
Carteolol 34
Carvedilol 34
Labetalol 34
Nadolol 34
Penbutolol 34
Pindolol 34
Propranolol 34
Sotalol 34
Timolol 34
Methadone
Amiodarone 83
Amprenavir 83
Atazanavir 83
Barbiturates 81
Bosentan 81
Carbamazepine 81
Cimetidine 83

Clarithromycin 82
Clotrimazole 82
Conivaptan 83
Cyclosporine 83
Darunavir 83
Delavirdine 83
Diltiazem 83
Efavirenz 81
Erythromycin 82
Fluconazole 82
Fluvoxamine 83
Grapefruit 83
Indinavir 83
Itraconazole 82
Ketoconazole 82
Nefazodone 83
Nelfinavir 83
Nevirapine 81
Oxcarbazepine 81
Phenytoin 81
Posaconazole 82
Primidone 81
Quinupristin 82
Ritonavir 83
Saquinavir 83
Telithromycin 82
Troleandomycin 82
Voriconazole 82
Rifampin 81
Rifapentine 81
Ritonavir 81
St. John's Wort 81
Verapamil 83
Methamphetamine.
  Amphetamines.
Methotrexate
Amoxicillin 84
Aspirin 84
Carbenicillin 84
Ciprofloxacin 84
Diclofenac 84
Diflunisal 84
Etodolac 84
Fenoprofen 84
Flurbiprofen 84
Ibuprofen 84
Indomethacin 84

<u>Underline</u> = Class 1;   *Italic* = Class 2;   Roman = Class 3

<u>Underline</u> = Class 1;   *Italic* = Class 2;   Roman = Class 3

Diflunisal 86
Etodolac 86
Fenoprofen 86
Fentanyl 83
Flurbiprofen 86
<u>Furazolidone</u> 78
Ibuprofen 86
Indomethacin 86
<u>Isocarboxazid</u> 78
Ketoprofen 86
Ketorolac 86
Linezolid 80
Meclofenamate 86
Mefenamic acid 86
Meloxicam 86
Meperidine 83
<u>Methylene Blue</u> 78
Nabumetone 86
Naproxen 86
Oxaprozin 86
<u>Phenelzine</u> 78
Piroxicam 86
Rasagiline 80
Selegiline 80
Sulindac 86
Thiazide Diuretics 104
Tolmetin 86
Tramadol 83
<u>Tranylcypromine</u> 78
Minocin. See Tetracyclines
Minocycline. See Tetracyclines
Mintezol. See Thiabendazole
Mirapex. See Pramipexole
Mirtazapine
  Clonidine 56
  <u>Furazolidone</u> 78
  <u>Isocarboxazid</u> 78
  Guanabenz 56
  Guanfacine 56
  Linezolid 80
  <u>Methylene Blue</u> 78
  <u>Phenelzine</u> 78
  Rasagiline 80
  Selegiline 80
  <u>Tranylcypromine</u> 78
Mobic. See Meloxicam

Moexipril. See ACE Inhibitors
Monistat. See Miconazole
Monopril. See ACE Inhibitors
Morphine
  Barbiturates 81
  Bosentan 81
  Carbamazepine 81
  Efavirenz 81
  Nevirapine 81
  Oxcarbazepine 81
  Phenytoin 81
  Primidone 81
  Rifampin 81
  Rifapentine 81
  St. John's Wort 81
Motrin. See Ibuprofen
Moxifloxacin. See also QTc table
  Antacids 95
  Calcium Polycarbophil 95
  Didanosine 95
  Iron 95
  Sucralfate 95
  Zinc 95
Multaq. See Dronedarone
Mycobutin. See Rifabutin
Mycophenolate
  Antacids 85
  Calcium Polycarbophil 85
  Cholestyramine 85
  Colestipol 85
  Iron 85
  Sucralfate 85
Mylanta. See Antacids
Mysoline. See Primidone
Nabumetone
  Acenocoumarol 31
  ACE Inhibitors 39
  Angiotensin Receptor Blockers 39
  Citalopram 86
  Clomipramine 86
  Duloxetine 86
  Escitalopram 86
  Fluoxetine 86

Fluvoxamine 86
Lithium 77
Methotrexate 84
Milnacipran 86
Nefazodone 86
Paroxetine 86
Phenprocoumon 31
Pralatrexate 84
Sertraline 86
Venlafaxine 86
Warfarin 31
Nadolol
  Chlorpropamide 34
  Epinephrine 49
  Glimepiride 34
  Glipizide 34
  Glyburide 34
  Insulin 34
  Metformin 34
  Nateglinide 34
  Pioglitazone 34
  Repaglinide 34
  Rosiglitazone 34
  Saxagliptin 34
  Tolbutamide 34
Nafcillin
  Acenocoumarol 27
  Amlodipine 51
  Bepridil 51
  Diltiazem 51
  Felodipine 51
  Isradipine 51
  Nicardipine 51
  Nifedipine 51
  Nimodipine 51
  Nisoldipine 51
  Nitrendipine 51
  Phenprocoumon 27
  Verapamil 51
  Warfarin 27
Nalfon. See Fenoprofen
Naproxen
  Acenocoumarol 31
  ACE Inhibitors 39
  Angiotensin Receptor Blockers 39
  Citalopram 86

<u>Underline</u> = Class 1;   *Italic* = Class 2;   Roman = Class 3

Clomipramine 86
Duloxetine 86
Escitalopram 86
Fluoxetine 86
Fluvoxamine 86
Lithium 77
Methotrexate 84
Milnacipran 86
Nefazodone 86
Paroxetine 86
Phenprocoumon 31
Pralatrexate 84
Sertraline 86
Venlafaxine 86
Warfarin 31
Naqua. See Thiazide
Diuretics
Naratriptan
  <u>Ergot Alkaloids</u> 70
Nardil. See Phenelzine
Nateglinide
  Amiodarone 36,38
  Amprenavir 38
  Aprepitant 38
  Atazanavir 38
  Capecitabine 36
  Carteolol 34
  Carvedilol 34
  Clarithromycin 36
  Conivaptan 38
  Co-trimoxazole 36
  Cyclosporine 38
  Darunavir 38
  Delavirdine 36,38
  Diltiazem 37
  Efavirenz 36
  Erythromycin 36
  Fluconazole 35
  Fluoxetine 36
  Fluorouracil 36
  Fluvastatin 36
  Fluvoxamine 36,38
  Grapefruit 38
  Indinavir 38
  Isoniazid 36
  Itraconazole 36
  Ketoconazole 36

Labetalol 34
Metronidazole 36
Nadolol 34
Nefazodone 38
Nelfinavir 38
Penbutolol 34
Pindolol 34
Posaconazole 36
Propranolol 34
Quinupristin 36
Ritonavir 38
Saquinavir 38
Sotalol 34
Sulfinpyrazone 36
Telithromycin 36
Timolol 34
Troleandomycin 36
Verapamil 37
Voriconazole 35
Naturetin. See Thiazide
Diuretics
Nebivolol
  Amiodarone 50
  Bupropion 49
  Cimetidine 50
  Cinacalcet 50
  Diphenhydramine 50
  Duloxetine 49
  Fluoxetine 49
  Haloperidol 50
  Paroxetine 49
  Propafenone 50
  Propoxyphene 50
  Quinidine 50
  Ritonavir 50
  Terbinafine 50
  Thioridazine 50
Nefazodone
  Alfentanil 83
  Alprazolam 40
  Amiodarone 23
  Amlodipine 51
  Amprenavir 91
  Antidepressants,
    tricyclic 33
  Aripiprazole 45
  Atazanavir 91

Atorvastatin 73
Bepridil 51
Buspirone 40
Carbamazepine 53
Clonazepam 40
Clorazepate 40
Colchicine 60
Corticosteroids 62
Cyclosporine 75
Darunavir 91
Dasatinib 107
Delavirdine 91
Diazepam 40
Diltiazem 51
Disopyramide 23
Dronedarone 23
Eplerenone 67
Ergot Alkaloids 68
Erlotinib 107
Estazolam 40
Fentanyl 83
Flurazepam 40
Gefitinib 107
Halazepam 40
Imatinib 107
Indinavir 91
Isradipine 51
Lapatinib 107
Lopinavir 91
Lovastatin 73
Methadone 83
Midazolam 40
Nateglinide 38
Nelfinavir 91
Nicardipine 51
Nifedipine 51
Nilotinib 107
Nimodipine 51
Nisoldipine 51
Nitrendipine 51
Oxycodone 83
Pazopanib 107
<u>Pimozide</u> 88
Pioglitazone 38
Prazepam 40
Quetiapine 94
Quinidine 23

<u>Underline</u> = Class 1;   *Italic* = Class 2;   Roman = Class 3

Ranolazine 96
Repaglinide 38
Rifabutin 97
Ritonavir 91
Saquinavir 91
Saxagliptin 38
Sildenafil 98
Simvastatin 73
Sirolimus 75
Sorafenib 107
Sufentanil 83
Sunitinib 107
Tacrolimus 75
Tadalafil 98
Tipranavir 91
Triazolam 40
Vardenafil 98
Verapamil 51
Vinblastine 111
Vincristine 111
Vinorelbine 111
Nelfinavir
Alfentanil 83
Alfuzosin 22
Alprazolam 43
Amiodarone 24, 92
Amlodipine 53
Amprenavir 92
Aprepitant 92
Aripiprazole 45
Atazanavir 92
Atorvastatin 73
Barbiturates 90
Bepridil 53
Bosentan 90
Buspirone 43
Carbamazepine 55,90
Clarithromycin 90
Clonazepam 43
Clorazepate 43
Colchicine 60
Conivaptan 92
Corticosteroids 63
Cyclosporine 75,92
Darunavir 92
Dasatinib 109
Delavirdine 92

Diazepam 43
Digoxin 65
Diltiazem 53,92
Disopyramide 24
Dronedarone 24
Efavirenz 90
Eplerenone 68
Ergot Alkaloids 70
Erlotinib 109
Erythromycin 90
Estazolam 43
Felodipine 53
Fentanyl 83
Fluconazole 90
Flurazepam 43
Fluvoxamine 91
Gefitinib 109
Grapefruit 92
Halazepam 43
Imatinib 109
Indinavir 92
Isradipine 53
Itraconazole 90
Ketoconazole 90
Lapatinib 109
Lopinavir 92
Lovastatin 73
Methadone 83
Midazolam 43
Nateglinide 38
Nefazodone 91
Nevirapine 90
Nicardipine 53
Nifedipine 53
Nilotinib 109
Nimodipine 53
Nisoldipine 53
Nitrendipine 53
Oxcarbazepine 90
Oxycodone 83
Pazopanib 109
Phenytoin 90
<u>Pimozide 88</u>
Pioglitazone 38
Posaconazole 90
Prazepam 43
Primidone 90

Quetiapine 94
Quinidine 24
Quinupristin 90
Ranolazine 96
Repaglinide 38
Rifabutin 90,98
Rifampin 90
Rifapentine 90
Ritonavir 92
Saquinavir 92
Saxagliptin 38
Sildenafil 100
Simvastatin 73
Sirolimus 75
Sorafenib 109
St. John's Wort 90
Sufentanil 83
Sunitinib 109
Tacrolimus 75
Tadalafil 100
Telithromycin 90
Tipranavir 92
Triazolam 43
Troleandomycin 90
Vardenafil 100
Verapamil 53,92
Vinblastine 111
Vincristine 111
Vinorelbine 111
Voriconazole 90
Nembutal. See Barbitur▸
Nevirapine. See also H▸
  Interaction chart
Amprenavir 90
Acetaminophen 21
Alfentanil 81
Amiodarone 24
Amlodipine 51
Antidepressants,
  tricyclic 32
Aripiprazole 43
Atazanavir 92
Atorvastatin 73
Bepridil 51
Contraceptives, oral
Corticosteroids 64
Cyclosporine 74

<u>Underline</u> = Class 1;   *Italic* = Class 2;   Roman = Class 3

<u>Underline</u> = Class 1;   *Italic* = Class 2;   Roman = Class 3

<u>Underline</u> = Class 1; *Italic* = Class 2; Roman = Class 3

Underline = Class 1;   *Italic* = Class 2;   Roman = Class 3

Ketoconazole 47
Lamotrigine 76
Lapatinib 109
Leflunomide 87
Lopinavir 90
Lovastatin 73
Methadone 81
Metronidazole 87
Morphine 81
Nelfinavir 90
Nicardipine 51
Nifedipine 51
Nilotinib 109
Nimodipine 51
Nisoldipine 51
Nitrendipine 51
Oxycodone 81
Pazopanib 109
Phenprocoumon 27
Quetiapine 92
Quinidine 24
Ritonavir 90
Saquinavir 90
Simvastatin 73
Sirolimus 74
Sorafenib 109
Sufentanil 81
Sulfamethoxazole 87
Sulfinpyrazone 87
Sunitinib 109
Tacrolimus 74
Theophylline 102
Ticlopidine 87
Tipranavir 90
Verapamil 51
Voriconazole 47,87
Warfarin 27
Zidovudine 112

Pimozide. See also QTc table
<u>Amiodarone</u> 88
<u>Amprenavir</u> 88
<u>Aprepitant</u> 88
<u>Atazanavir</u> 88
<u>Clarithromycin</u> 87
<u>Conivaptan</u> 88
<u>Cyclosporine</u> 88
<u>Darunavir</u> 88

<u>Delavirdine</u> 88
<u>Diltiazem</u> 88
<u>Erythromycin</u> 87
<u>Fluconazole</u> 87
<u>Fluvoxamine</u> 88
<u>Grapefruit</u> 88
<u>Indinavir</u> 88
<u>Itraconazole</u> 87
<u>Ketoconazole</u> 87
<u>Nefazodone</u> 88
<u>Nelfinavir</u> 88
<u>Paroxetine</u> 88
<u>Posaconazole</u> 87
<u>Quinupristin</u> 87
<u>Ritonavir</u> 88
<u>Saquinavir</u> 88
<u>Sertraline</u> 88
<u>Telithromycin</u> 87
<u>Troleandomycin</u> 87
<u>Verapamil</u> 88
<u>Voriconazole</u> 87

Pindolol
Chlorpropamide 34
Epinephrine 49
Glimepiride 34
Glipizide 34
Glyburide 34
Insulin 34
Metformin 34
Nateglinide 34
Pioglitazone 34
Rosiglitazone 34
Repaglinide 34
Saxagliptin 34
Tolbutamide 34

Pioglitazone
Amiodarone 38
Amprenavir 38
Aprepitant 38
Atazanavir 38
Carteolol 34
Carvedilol 34
Clarithromycin 36
Conivaptan 38
Cyclosporine 38
Darunavir 38
Delavirdine 38

Diltiazem 37
Erythromycin 36
Fluconazole 36
Fluvoxamine 36
Grapefruit 38
Indinavir 38
Isoniazid 36
Itraconazole 36
Ketoconazole 36
Labetalol 34
Nadolol 34
Nefazodone 38
Nelfinavir 38
Penbutolol 34
Pindolol 34
Posaconazole 36
Propranolol 34
Quinupristin 36
Ritonavir 38
Saquinavir 38
Sotalol 34
Telithromycin 36
Timolol 34
Troleandomycin 36
Verapamil 37
Voriconazole 36

Piperacillin
Methotrexate 84

Piroxicam
Acenocoumarol 31
ACE Inhibitors 39
Angiotensin Receptor
  Blockers 39
Citalopram 86
Clomipramine 86
Duloxetine 86
Escitalopram 86
Fluoxetine 86
Fluvoxamine 86
Lithium 77
Methotrexate 84
Milnacipran 86
Nefazodone 86
Paroxetine 86
Phenprocoumon 31
Sertraline 86
Venlafaxine 86

<u>Underline</u> = Class 1;   *Italic* = Class 2;   Roman = Class 3

Warfarin 31
Plendil. See Felodipine
Polythiazide. See Thiazide
  Diuretics
Posaconazole
  Alfentanil 82
  Alfuzosin 21
  Alprazolam 41
  Amiodarone 22
  Amlodipine 52
  Amprenavir 90
  Aripiprazole 44
  Atazanavir 90
  Atorvastatin 71
  Barbiturates 47
  Bepridil 52
  Budesonide 62
  Buspirone 41
  Calcium channel
    blockers 52
  Carbamazepine 47,54
  Clonazepam 41
  Clorazepate 41
  Colchicine 59
  Corticosteroids 62
  Cyclosporine 75
  Darunavir 90
  Dasatinib 108
  Delavirdine 90
  Dexamethasone 62
  Diazepam 41
  Digoxin 65
  Diltiazem 41
  Disopyramide 22
  Dronedarone 22
  Efavirenz 47
  Eplerenone 67
  Ergot Alkaloids 69
  Erlotinib 108
  Estazolam 41
  Felodipine 52
  Fentanyl 82
  Flurazepam 41
  Fluticasone 62
  Gefitinib 108
  Halazepam 41
  Imatinib 108

Indinavir 90
Isradipine 52
Lapatinib 108
Lopinavir 90
Lovastatin 71
Methadone 82
Methylprednisolone 62
Midazolam 41
Nateglinide 36
Nelfinavir 90
Nevirapine 47
Nicardipine 52
Nifedipine 52
Nilotinib 108
Nimodipine 52
Nisoldipine 52
Nitrendipine 52
Oxcarbazepine 47
Oxycodone 82
Pazopanib 108
Phenytoin 47
<u>Pimozide</u> 87
Pioglitazone 36
Prazepam 41
Primidone 47
Quetiapine 93
Quinidine 22
Ranolazine 95
Repaglinide 36
Rifabutin 47,97
Rifampin 47
Rifapentine 47
Ritonavir 90
Saquinavir 90
Saxagliptin 36
Sildenafil 99
Simvastatin 71
Sirolimus 75
Sorafenib 108
St. John's Wort 47
Sufentanil 82
Sunitinib 108
Tacrolimus 75
Tadalafil 99
Tipranavir 90
Triazolam 41
Vardenafil 99

Verapamil 52
Vinblastine 110
Vincristine 110
Vinorelbine 110
Potassium-sparing diu
  ACE inhibitors 89
  Potassium 89
Potassium
  ACE inhibitors 89
  Potassium-sparing
    diuretics 89
Pralatrexate
  Amoxicillin 84
  Aspirin 84
  Carbenicillin 84
  Ciprofloxacin 84
  Diclofenac 84
  Diflunisal 84
  Etodolac 84
  Fenoprofen 84
  Flurbiprofen 84
  Ibuprofen 84
  Indomethacin 84
  Ketoprofen 84
  Ketorolac 84
  Meclofenamate 84
  Mefenamic acid 84
  Meloxicam 84
  Mezlocillin 84
  Nabumetone 84
  Naproxen 84
  Omeprazole 84
  Oxacillin 84
  Oxaprozin 84
  Pantoprazole 84
  Penicillins 84
  Piperacillin 84
  Piroxicam 84
  Probenecid 84
  Salicylates 84
  Sulindac 84
  Thiazide Diuretics 84
  Tolmetin 84
  Trimethoprim 84
Pramipexole
  Haloperidol 66
  Metoclopramide 66

<u>Underline</u> = Class 1;   *Italic* = Class 2;   Roman = Class 3

Underline = Class 1;   *Italic* = Class 2;   Roman = Class 3

Fluoxetine 25
Haloperidol 25
Hydrocodone 58
Metoprolol 50
Mexiletine 25
Nebivolol 50
Paroxetine 25
Propoxyphene 25
Propranolol 50
Quinidine 25
Ritonavir 25
Tamoxifen 101
Terbinafine 25
Timolol 50
<u>Thioridazine</u> 25,104
Warfarin 31
Propoxyphene
  Antidepressants,
    tricyclic 34
  Aripiprazole 46
  Carbamazepine 55
  Carvedilol 50
  Codeine 58
  Dihydrocodeine 58
  Flecainide 25
  <u>Furazolidone</u> 78
  Hydrocodone 58
  <u>Isocarboxazid</u> 78
  Linezolid 80
  <u>Methylene Blue</u> 78
  Metoprolol 50
  Mexiletine 25
  Nebivolol 50
  <u>Phenelzine</u> 78
  Propafenone 25
  Propranolol 50
  Rasagiline 80
  Selegiline 80
  Tamoxifen 101
  Thioridazine 105
  Timolol 50
  <u>Tranylcypromine</u> 78
Propranolol
  Amiodarone 50
  Bupropion 49
  Chlorpropamide 34
  Cimetidine 50

Cinacalcet 50
Diphenhydramine 50
Duloxetine 49
Epinephrine 49
Fluoxetine 49
Glimepiride 34
Glipizide 34
Glyburide 34
Haloperidol 50
Insulin 34
Metformin 34
Nateglinide 34
Paroxetine 49
Pioglitazone 34
Propafenone 50
Propoxyphene 50
Quinidine 50
Repaglinide 34
Ritonavir 50
Rosiglitazone 34
Saxagliptin 34
Terbinafine 50
Thioridazine 50
Tolbutamide 34
Protonix. See Pantoprazole
Protriptyline. See
  Antidepressants, tricyclic
Prozac. See Fluoxetine
Pseudoephedrine
  <u>Furazolidone</u> 79
  <u>Isocarboxazid</u> 79
  <u>Linezolid</u> 81
  <u>Methylene Blue</u> 79
  <u>Phenelzine</u> 79
  Rasagiline 81
  Selegiline 81
  <u>Tranylcypromine</u> 79
Purinethol. See
  Mercaptopurine
Questran. See
  Cholestyramine
Quetiapine
  Amiodarone 94
  Amprenavir 94
  Aprepitant 94
  Atazanavir 94
  Barbiturates 92

Bosentan 92
Carbamazepine 92
Clarithromycin 93
Conivaptan 94
Cyclosporine 94
Darunavir 94
Delavirdine 94
Diltiazem 94
Efavirenz 92
Erythromycin 93
Fluconazole 93
Fluvoxamine 94
Grapefruit 94
Indinavir 94
Itraconazole 93
Ketoconazole 93
Nefazodone 94
Nelfinavir 94
Nevirapine 92
Oxcarbazepine 92
Phenobarbital 92
Phenytoin 92
Posaconazole 93
Primidone 92
Quinupristin 93
Rifabutin 92
Rifampin 92
Rifapentine 92
Ritonavir 94
Saquinavir 94
St. John's Wort 92
Telithromycin 93
Troleandomycin 93
Verapamil 94
Voriconazole 93
Quilinggao. See Herbal
  Interaction chart
Quinaglute. See Quinidi\~
Quinalan. See Quinidine
Quinidex. See Quinidine
Quinapril. See ACE
  Inhibitors
Quinethazone. See Thia\~
  Diuretics
Quinidine. See also QT
  table
  Amiodarone 24

<u>Underline</u> = Class 1;   *Italic* = Class 2;   Roman = Class 3

Amprenavir 24
Antidepressants, tricyclic 34
Aprepitant 24
Aripiprazole 46
Atazanavir 24
Barbiturates 24
Carbamazepine 24
Carvedilol 50
Clarithromycin 22
Codeine 58
Colchicine 60
Conivaptan 24
Cyclosporine 24
Darunavir 24
Delavirdine 24
Digoxin 65
Dihydrocodeine 58
Diltiazem 23
Efavirenz 24
Erythromycin 22
Flecainide 25
Fluconazole 22
Fluvoxamine 23
Grapefruit 24
Hydrocodone 58
Indinavir 24
Itraconazole 22
Ketoconazole 22
Metoprolol 50
Mexiletine 25
Nebivolol 50
Nefazodone 23
Nelfinavir 24
Nevirapine 24
Oxcarbazepine 24
Phenytoin 24
Posaconazole 22
Primidone 24
Propafenone 36
Propranolol 50
Quinupristin 22
Rifabutin 24
Rifampin 24
Rifapentine 24
Ritonavir 24
St. John's Wort 24

Saquinavir 24
Tamoxifen 101
Telithromycin 22
<u>Thioridazine</u> 104
Timolol 50
Troleandomycin 22
Verapamil 23
Voriconazole 22
Quinolones. See individual agents
Quinupristin
Alfentanil 82
Alfuzosin 21
Alprazolam 41
Amiodarone 22
Amlodipine 52
Amprenavir 90
Aripiprazole 44
Atazanavir 90
Atorvastatin 71
Bepridil 52
Buspirone 41
Carbamazepine 54
Clonazepam 41
Clorazepate 41
Colchicine 59
Cyclosporine 75
Darunavir 90
Dasatinib 108
Delavirdine 90
Diazepam 42
Diltiazem 52
Disopyramide 22
Dronedarone 22
Eplerenone 67
Ergot Alkaloids 69
Erlotinib 108
Estazolam 41
Felodipine 52
Fentanyl 82
Flurazepam 41
Gefitinib 108
Halazepam 41
Imatinib 108
Indinavir 90
Isradipine 52
Lapatinib 108

Lopinavir 90
Lovastatin 71
Methadone 82
Midazolam 41
Nateglinide 36
Nelfinavir 90
Nicardipine 52
Nifedipine 52
Nilotinib 108
Nimodipine 52
Nisoldipine 52
Nitrendipine 52
Oxycodone 82
Pazopanib 108
<u>Pimozide</u> 87
Pioglitazone 36
Prazepam 41
Quetiapine 93
Quinidine 22
Ranolazine 95
Repaglinide 36
Rifabutin 97
Ritonavir 90
Saquinavir 90
Saxagliptin 36
Sildenafil 99
Simvastatin 71
Sirolimus 75
Sorafenib 108
Sufentanil 82
Sunitinib 108
Tacrolimus 75
Tadalafil 99
Tipranavir 90
Triazolam 41
Vardenafil 99
Verapamil 52
Vinblastine 110
Vincristine 110
Vinorelbine 110
Rabeprazole
Cefditoren 56
Cefpodoxime 56
Cefuroxime 56
Glipizide 38
Glyburide 38
Itraconazole 48

<u>Underline</u> = Class 1;   *Italic* = Class 2;   Roman = Class 3

<u>Underline</u> = Class 1;   *Italic* = Class 2;   Roman = Class 3

<u>Underline</u> = Class 1;   *Italic* = Class 2;   Roman = Class 3

Underline = Class 1;   *Italic* = Class 2;   Roman = Class 3

Indinavir 92
Isradipine 53
Itraconazole 90
Ketoconazole 90
Lapatinib 109
Lopinavir 92
Lovastatin 73
Methadone 83
Midazolam 43
Nateglinide 38
Nefazodone 91
Nelfinavir 92
Nevirapine 90
Nicardipine 53
Nifedipine 53
Nilotinib 109
Nimodipine 53
Nisoldipine 53
Nitrendipine 53
Oxcarbazepine 90
Oxycodone 83
Pazopanib 109
Phenytoin 90
Pimozide 88
Pioglitazone 38
Posaconazole 90
Prazepam 43
Primidone 90
Quetiapine 94
Quinidine 24
Quinupristin 90
Ranolazine 96
Repaglinide 38
Rifabutin 90,98
Rifampin 90
Rifapentine 90
Ritonavir 92
Saxagliptin 38
Sildenafil 100
Simvastatin 73
Sirolimus 75
Sorafenib 109
St. John's Wort 90
Sufentanil 83
Sunitinib 109
Tacrolimus 75
Tadalafil 100

Telithromycin 90
Tipranavir 92
Triazolam 43
Troleandomycin 90
Vardenafil 100
Verapamil 53,92
Vinblastine 111
Vincristine 111
Vinorelbine 111
Voriconazole 90
Savella. See Milnacipran
Saxagliptin
  Amiodarone 38
  Amprenavir 38
  Aprepitant 38
  Atazanavir 38
  Carteolol 34
  Carvedilol 34
  Clarithromycin 36
  Conivaptan 38
  Cyclosporine 38
  Darunavir 38
  Delavirdine 38
  Diltiazem 36
  Erythromycin 36
  Fluconazole 36
  Fluvoxamine 38
  Grapefruit 38
  Indinavir 38
  Isoniazid 36
  Itraconazole 36
  Ketoconazole 36
  Labetalol 34
  Nadolol 34
  Nefazodone 38
  Nelfinavir 38
  Penbutolol 34
  Pindolol 34
  Posaconazole 36
  Propranolol 34
  Quinupristin 36
  Ritonavir 38
  Saquinavir 38
  Sotalol 34
  Telithromycin 36
  Timolol 34
  Troleandomycin 36

Verapamil 36
Voriconazole 36
Secobarbital. See
  Barbiturates
Selegiline. See MAO-B
  Inhibitors
Sensipar. See Cinacalcet
Septra. See Sulfamethoxa
Serentil. See Phenothiazir
Seroquel. See Quetiapine
Sertraline
  Diclofenac 86
  Diflunisal 86
  Etodolac 86
  Fenoprofen 86
  Flurbiprofen 86
  Furazolidone 78
  Ibuprofen 86
  Indomethacin 86
  Isocarboxazid 78
  Ketoprofen 86
  Ketorolac 86
  Linezolid 80
  Meclofenamate 86
  Mefenamic acid 86
  Meloxicam 86
  Meperidine 83
  Methylene Blue 78
  Naproxen 86
  Oxaprozin 86
  Phenelzine 78
  Pimozide 68
  Piroxicam 86
  Rasagiline 80
  Selegiline 80
  Sulindac 86
  Thiazide Diuretics 104
  Tolmetin 86
  Tramadol 83
  Tranylcypromine 78
Sevelamer
  Thyroid 106
Sibutramine
  Furazolidone 78
  Isocarboxazid 78
  Linezolid 80
  Methylene Blue 78

Underline = Class 1;   *Italic* = Class 2;   Roman = Class 3

180

Phenelzine 78
Rasagiline 80
Selegiline 80
Tranylcypromine 78
Sildenafil
Amiodarone 100
Amprenavir 100
Aprepitant 100
Atazanavir 100
Cimetidine 100
Clarithromycin 99
Conivaptan 100
Cyclosporine 100
Darunavir 100
Delavirdine 100
Diltiazem 99
Erythromycin 99
Fluconazole 99
Fluvoxamine 98
Grapefruit 100
Indinavir 100
Isosorbide dinitrate 85
Itraconazole 99
Ketoconazole 99
Nefazodone 98
Nelfinavir 100
Nitrates 85
Nitroglycerin 85
Posaconazole 99
Quinupristin 99
Ritonavir 100
Saquinavir 100
Telithromycin 99
Troleandomycin 99
Verapamil 99
Voriconazole 99
Simvastatin
Acenocoumarol 28
Amiodarone 73
Amprenavir 73
Atazanavir 73
Barbiturates 73
Carbamazepine 73
Clarithromycin 71
Conivaptan 73
Cyclosporine 73
Darunavir 73

Delavirdine 73
Diltiazem 71
Efavirenz 73
Erythromycin 71
Etravirine 73
Fluconazole 71
Fluvoxamine 71
Gemfibrozil 72
Grapefruit 73
Imatinib 73
Indinavir 73
Itraconazole 71
Ketoconazole 71
Nefazodone 73
Nelfinavir 73
Nevirapine 73
Oxcarbazepine 73
Phenytoin 73
Posaconazole 71
Primidone 73
Quinupristin 71
Rifabutin 73
Rifampin 73
Rifapentine 73
Ritonavir 73
St. John's Wort 73
Saquinavir 73
Telithromycin 71
Troleandomycin 71
Verapamil 71
Voriconazole 71
Warfarin 28
Sinequan. See Antidepres-
sants, tricyclic
Sirolimus
Amiodarone 75
Amprenavir 75
Androgens 75
Aprepitant 75
Atazanavir 75
Azithromycin 75
Barbiturates 74
Bosentan 74
Carbamazepine 74
Chloroquine 75
Clarithromycin 75
Clotrimazole 75

Conivaptan 75
Contraceptives, oral 75
Danazol 75
Darunavir 75
Delavirdine 75
Diltiazem 75
Efavirenz 74
Erythromycin 75
Fluconazole 75
Fluvoxamine 75
Grapefruit 75
Indinavir 75
Itraconazole 75
Ketoconazole 75
Levothyroxine 74
Methoxsalen 75
Nefazodone 75
Nelfinavir 75
Nevirapine 74
Nicardipine 75
Oxcarbazepine 74
Phenytoin 74
Posaconazole 75
Primidone 74
Quinupristin 75
Rifabutin 74
Rifampin 74
Rifapentine 74
Ritonavir 75
St. John's Wort 74
Saquinavir 75
Telithromycin 75
Troleandomycin 75
Verapamil 75
Voriconazole 75
Slo-bid. See Theophylline
Slo-Phyllin. See
Theophylline
Sorafenib
Amiodarone 109
Amprenavir 109
Aprepitant 109
Atazanavir 109
Barbiturates 109
Carbamazepine 109
Clarithromycin 108
Conivaptan 109

<u>Underline</u> = Class 1;   *Italic* = Class 2;   Roman = Class 3

<u>Underline</u> = Class 1;   *Italic* = Class 2;   Roman = Class 3

ACE Inhibitors 39
Angiotensin Receptor
  Blockers 39
Citalopram 86
Clomipramine 86
Duloxetine 86
Escitalopram 86
Fluoxetine 86
Fluvoxamine 86
Lithium 77
Methotrexate 84
Milnacipran 86
Nefazodone 86
Paroxetine 86
Phenprocoumon 31
Pralatrexate 84
Sertraline 86
Venlafaxine 86
Warfarin 31

Sumatriptan. See also QTc
table
  <u>Ergot Alkaloids</u> 70

Sunitinib
  Amiodarone 109
  Amprenavir 109
  Aprepitant 109
  Atazanavir 109
  Barbiturates 109
  Carbamazepine 109
  Clarithromycin 108
  Conivaptan 109
  Cyclosporine 109
  Darunavir 109
  Delavirdine 109
  Diltiazem 109
  Efavirenz 109
  Erythromycin 108
  Fluconazole 108
  Fluvoxamine 107
  Grapefruit 109
  Indinavir 109
  Isoniazid 108
  Itraconazole 108
  Ketoconazole 108
  Nefazodone 107
  Nelfinavir 109
  Nevirapine 109

Oxcarbazepine 109
Phenytoin 109
Posaconazole 108
Primidone 109
Quinupristin 108
Rifabutin 109
Rifampin 109
Rifapentine 109
Ritonavir 109
Saquinavir 109
St. John's Wort 109
Telithromycin 108
Troleandomycin 108
Verapamil 109
Voriconazole 108
Surmontil. See
  Antidepressants, tricyclic
Sutent. See Sunitinib
Sympathomimetics. See
  individual agents
Synalgos-DC. See
  Dihydrocodeine
Synthroid. See Thyroid

Tacrine
  Clozapine 57
  Olanzapine 57
  Theophylline 103
  Tizanidine 106

Tacrolimus
  Amiodarone 75
  Amprenavir 75
  Androgens 75
  Aprepitant 75
  Atazanavir 75
  Azithromycin 75
  Barbiturates 74
  Bosentan 74
  Carbamazepine 74
  Chloroquine 75
  Clarithromycin 75
  Clotrimazole 75
  Colchicine 60
  Conivaptan 75
  Contraceptives, oral 75
  Danazol 75
  Darunavir 75
  Delavirdine 75

Digoxin 65
Diltiazem 75
Efavirenz 74
Erythromycin 75
Fluconazole 75
Fluvoxamine 75
Grapefruit 75
Indinavir 75
Itraconazole 75
Ketoconazole 75
Levothyroxine 74
Methoxsalen 75
Nefazodone 75
Nelfinavir 75
Nevirapine 74
Nicardipine 75
Oxcarbazepine 74
Phenytoin 75
Posaconazole 75
Primidone 74
Quinupristin 75
Rifabutin 74
Rifampin 74
Rifapentine 74
Ritonavir 75
Saquinavir 75
St. John's Wort 74
Telithromycin 75
Troleandomycin 75
Verapamil 75
Voriconazole 75

Tadalafil
  Amiodarone 100
  Amprenavir 100
  Aprepitant 100
  Atazanavir 100
  Cimetidine 100
  Clarithromycin 99
  Conivaptan 100
  Cyclosporine 100
  Darunavir 100
  Delavirdine 100
  Diltiazem 99
  Erythromycin 99
  Fluconazole 99
  Fluvoxamine 98
  Grapefruit 100

<u>Underline</u> = Class 1;   *Italic* = Class 2;   Roman = Class 3

Indinavir 100
Itraconazole 99
Ketoconazole 99
Nefazodone 98
Nelfinavir 100
<u>Nitrates</u> 85
Posaconazole 99
Quinupristin 99
Ritonavir 100
Saquinavir 100
Telithromycin 99
Troleandomycin 99
Verapamil 99
Voriconazole 99
Tagamet. See Cimetidine
Tambocor. See Flecainide
Tamoxifen
  Acenocoumarol 31
  Amiodarone 101
  Bupropion 100
  Cimetidine 101
  Cinacalcet 101
  Colchicine 60
  Diphenhydramine 101
  Duloxetine 100
  Digoxin 65
  Fluoxetine 100
  Haloperidol 101
  Paroxetine 100
  Propafenone 101
  Propoxyphene 101
  Quinidine 101
  Ritonavir 101
  Terbinafine 101
  Thioridazine 101
  Warfarin 31
TAO. See Troleandomycin
Tapentadol
  <u>Furazolidone</u> 79
  <u>Isocarboxazid</u> 79
  <u>Linezolid</u> 81
  <u>Methylene Blue</u> 79
  <u>Phenelzine</u> 81
  Rasagiline 81
  Selegiline 81
  <u>Tranylcypromine</u> 79
Tarceva. See Erlotinib

Tarka. See ACE Inhibitors
  and calcium channel
  blockers
Tasigna. See Nilotinib
Tegretol. See Carbamazepine
Telithromycin
  Alfentanil 82
  Alfuzosin 21
  Alprazolam 41
  Amiodarone 22
  Amlodipine 52
  Amprenavir 90
  Aripiprazole 44
  Atazanavir 90
  Atorvastatin 71
  Bepridil 52
  Budesonide 62
  Buspirone 41
  Carbamazepine 54
  Clonazepam 41
  Clorazepate 41
  Colchicine 59
  Cyclosporine 75
  Darunavir 90
  Dasatinib 108
  Delavirdine 90
  Dexamethasone 62
  Diazepam 41
  Digoxin 65
  Diltiazem 52
  Disopyramide 22
  Dronedarone 22
  Eplerenone 67
  Ergot Alkaloids 69
  Erlotinib 108
  Estazolam 41
  Felodipine 52
  Fentanyl 82
  Flurazepam 41
  Fluticasone 62
  Gefitinib 108
  Halazepam 41
  Imatinib 108
  Indinavir 90
  Isradipine 52
  Lapatinib 108
  Lopinavir 90

Lovastatin 71
Methadone 82
Methylprednisolone 62
Midazolam 41
Nateglinide 36
Nelfinavir 90
Nicardipine 52
Nifedipine 52
Nilotinib 108
Nimodipine 52
Nisoldipine 52
Nitrendipine 52
Oxycodone 82
Pazopanib 108
<u>Pimozide</u> 87
Pioglitazone 36
Prazepam 41
Quetiapine 93
Quinidine 22
Ranolazine 95
Repaglinide 36
Rifabutin 97
Ritonavir 90
Saquinavir 90
Saxagliptin 36
Sildenafil 99
Simvastatin 71
Sirolimus 75
Sorafenib 108
Sufentanil 82
Sunitinib 108
Tacrolimus 75
Tadalafil 99
Tipranavir 90
Triazolam 41
Vardenafil 99
Verapamil 52
Vinblastine 110
Vincristine 110
Vinorelbine 110
Telmisartan. See Angioter
  Receptor Blockers
Tenuate. See Diethylpropi
Terbinafine
  Antidepressants,
    tricyclic 34
  Aripiprazole 46

<u>Underline</u> = Class 1;   *Italic* = Class 2;   Roman = Class 3

<u>Underline</u> = Class 1; *Italic* = Class 2; Roman = Class 3

Ticlid. See Ticlopidine
Ticlopidine
  Phenytoin 87
  Theophylline 103
Timolol
  Amiodarone 50
  Bupropion 49
  Chlorpropamide 34
  Cimetidine 50
  Cinacalcet 50
  Diphenhydramine 50
  Duloxetine 49
  Epinephrine 49
  Fluoxetine 49
  Glimepiride 34
  Glipizide 34
  Glyburide 34
  Haloperidol 50
  Insulin 34
  Metformin 34
  Nateglinide 34
  Paroxetine 49
  Pioglitazone 34
  Propafenone 50
  Propoxyphene 50
  Quinidine 50
  Repaglinide 34
  Ritonavir 50
  Rosiglitazone 34
  Terbinafine 50
  Saxagliptin 34
  Thioridazine 50
  Tolbutamide 34
Tipranavir
  Amiodarone 92
  Amprenavir 92
  Aprepitant 92
  Atazanavir 92
  Barbiturates 90
  Bosentan 90
  Carbamazepine 90
  Clarithromycin 90
  Conivaptan 92
  Cyclosporine 92
  Darunavir 92
  Delavirdine 92
  Diltiazem 92

Efavirenz 90
Erythromycin 90
Fluconazole 90
Fluvoxamine 91
Grapefruit 92
Indinavir 92
Itraconazole 90
Ketoconazole 90
Nefazodone 91
Nelfinavir 92
Nevirapine 90
Oxcarbamazepine 90
Phenytoin 90
Posaconazole 90
Primidone 90
Quinupristin 90
Rifabutin 90
Rifampin 90
Rifapentine 90
Ritonavir 92
St. John's Wort 90
Saquinavir 92
Telithromycin 90
Troleandomycin 90
Verapamil 92
Voriconazole 90
Tizanidine
  Atazanavir 106
  Cimetidine 106
  Ciprofloxacin 106
  Enoxacin 106
  Fluvoxamine 106
  Mexiletine 106
  Tacrine 106
  Zileuton 106
Tofranil. See Imipramine
Tolbutamide
  Amiodarone 36
  Capecitabine 36
  Carteolol 34
  Carvedilol 34
  Delavirdine 36
  Efavirenz 36
  Fluconazole 35
  Fluoxetine 36
  Fluorouracil 36
  Fluvastatin 36

Fluvoxamine 36
Labetalol 34
Metronidazole 36
Nadolol 34
Penbutolol 34
Pindolol 34
Propranolol 34
Sotalol 34
Sulfinpyrazone 36
Timolol 34
Voriconazole 35
Tolectin. See Tolmetin
Tolmetin
  Acenocoumarol 31
  ACE Inhibitors 39
  Angiotensin Receptor
    Blockers 39
  Citalopram 86
  Clomipramine 86
  Duloxetine 86
  Escitalopram 86
  Fluoxetine 86
  Fluvoxamine 86
  Lithium 77
  Methotrexate 84
  Milnacipran 86
  Nefazodone 86
  Paroxetine 86
  Phenprocoumon 31
  Pralatrexate 84
  Sertraline 86
  Venlafaxine 86
  Warfarin 31
Topamax. See Topiramat
Topiramate
  Contraceptives, oral 6▮
  Corticosteroids
Toradol. See Ketorolac
Torsemide
  Cholestyramine 65
  Colestipol 65
  Lithium 77
Tramadol
  Citalopram 83
  Clomipramine 83
  Desvenlafaxine 83
  Duloxetine 83

<u>Underline</u> = Class 1;   *Italic* = Class 2;   Roman = Class 3

Underline = Class 1; *Italic* = Class 2; Roman = Class 3

Nitrendipine 52
Oxycodone 82
Pazopanib 108
Pimozide 87
Pioglitazone 36
Prazepam 41
Quetiapine 93
Quinidine 22
Ranolazine 95
Repaglinide 36
Rifabutin 97
Ritonavir 90
Saquinavir 90
Saxagliptin 36
Sildenafil 99
Simvastatin 71
Sirolimus 75
Sorafenib 108
Sufentanil 82
Sunitinib 108
Tacrolimus 75
Tadalafil 99
Theophylline 103
Tipranavir 90
Triazolam 41
Vardenafil 99
Verapamil 52
Vinblastine 110
Vincristine 110
Vinorelbine 110
Tums. See Antacids
Tykerb. See Lapatinib
Tylenol. See Acetaminophen
Uloric. See Febuxostat
Ultram. See Tramadol
Uni-Dur. See Theophylline
Unipen. See Nafcillin
Univasc. See ACE Inhibitors
Urobiotic. See
  Sulfamethizole
Uroxatral. See Alfuzosin
Valdecoxib
  Lithium 77
Valerain. See Herbal
  Interaction chart
Valium. See Diazepam
Valproic Acid

Ertapenem 110
Imipenem 110
Lamotrigine 76
Meropenem 110
Zidovudine 112
Valsartan. See Angiotensin
  Receptor Blockers
Vantin. See Cefpodoxime
Vaprisol. See Conivaptan
Vardenafil
  Amiodarone 100
  Amprenavir 100
  Aprepitant 100
  Atazanavir 100
  Cimetidine 100
  Clarithromycin 99
  Conivaptan 100
  Cyclosporine 100
  Darunavir 100
  Delavirdine 100
  Diltiazem 99
  Erythromycin 99
  Fluconazole 99
  Fluvoxamine 98
  Grapefruit 100
  Indinavir 100
  Isosorbide dinitrate 85
  Itraconazole 99
  Ketoconazole 99
  Nefazodone 98
  Nelfinavir 100
  Nitrates 85
  Nitroglycerin 85
  Posaconazole 99
  Quinupristin 99
  Ritonavir 100
  Saquinavir 100
  Telithromycin 99
  Troleandomycin 99
  Verapamil 99
  Voriconazole 99
Vascor. See Bepridil
Vasotec. See ACE Inhibitors
Velban. See Vinblastine
Venlafaxine
  Diclofenac 86
  Diflunisal 86

Etodolac 86
Fenoprofen 7
Flurbiprofen 86
Furazolidone 78
Ibuprofen 86
Indomethacin 86
Isocarboxazid 78
Ketoprofen 86
Ketorolac 86
Linezolid 80
Meclofenamate 86
Mefenamic acid 86
Meloxicam 86
Meperidine 83
Methylene Blue 78
Nabumetone 86
Naproxen 86
Oxaprozin 86
Phenelzine 78
Piroxicam 86
Rasagiline 80
Selegiline 80
Sulindac 86
Thiazide Diuretics 104
Tolmetin 86
Tramadol 83
Tranylcypromine 78
Verapamil. See also Calc
  channel blockers
See also Herbal Interactic
  chart
  Alfentanil 83
  Alfuzosin 22
  Alprazolam 42
  Amiodarone 23
  Amlodipine 53
  Amprenavir 92
  Aripiprazole 45
  Atazanavir 92
  Atorvastatin 71
  Bepridil 53
  Budesonide 63
  Buspirone 42
  Carbamazepine 54
  Clonazepam 42
  Clorazepate 42
  Colchicine 60

Underline = Class 1;   *Italic* = Class 2;   Roman = Class 3

Corticosteroids 63
Cyclosporine 75
Darunavir 92
Dasatinib 109
Delavirdine 92
Dexamethasone 63
Diazepam 42
Digoxin 64
Diltiazem 53
Disopyramide 23
Dronedarone 23
Eplerenone 68
Ergot Alkaloids 70
Erlotinib 109
Estazolam 42
Felodipine 53
Fentanyl 83
Fluticasone 63
Flurazepam 42
Fluvoxamine 51
Gefitinib 109
Halazepam 42
Imatinib 109
Indinavir 92
Isradipine 53
Lapatinib 109
Lopinavir 92
Lovastatin 71
Methadone 83
Methylprednisolone 63
Midazolam 42
Nateglinide 37
Nefazodone 51
Nelfinavir 92
Nicardipine 53
Nifedipine 53
Nilotinib 109
Nimodipine 53
Nisoldipine 53
Nitrendipine 53
Oxycodone 83
Pazopanib 109
<u>Pimozide</u> 88
Pioglitazone 37
Prazepam 42
Quetiapine 94
Quinidine 23

Ranolazine 96
Repaglinide 37
Rifabutin 51,98
Ritonavir 92
Saquinavir 92
Saxagliptin 37
Sildenafil 99
Simvastatin 71
Sirolimus 75
Sorafenib 109
Sufentanil 83
Sunitinib 109
Tacrolimus 75
Tadalafil 99
Tipranavir 92
Triazolam 42
Vardenafil 99
Vinblastine 111
Vincristine 111
Vinorelbine 111
Versed. See Midazolam
Viagra. See Sildenafil
Vibramycin. See
 Tetracyclines
Vicodin. See Hydrocodone
Videx. See Didanosine
Vinblastine
Amiodarone 111
Amprenavir 111
Aprepitant 111
Atazanavir 111
Clarithromycin 110
Conivaptan 111
Cyclosporine 111
Darunavir 111
Delavirdine 111
Diltiazem 111
Erythromycin 110
Fluconazole 110
Fluvoxamine 111
Grapefruit 111
Indinavir 111
Itraconazole 110
Ketoconazole 110
Nefazodone 111
Nelfinavir 111
Nicardipine 111

Nifedipine 111
Posaconazole 110
Quinupristin 110
Ritonavir 111
Saquinavir 111
Telithromycin 110
Troleandomycin 110
Verapamil 111
Voriconazole 110
Vincristine
Amiodarone 111
Amprenavir 111
Aprepitant 111
Atazanavir 111
Clarithromycin 110
Conivaptan 111
Cyclosporine 111
Darunavir 111
Delavirdine 111
Diltiazem 111
Erythromycin 110
Fluconazole 110
Fluvoxamine 111
Grapefruit 111
Indinavir 111
Itraconazole 110
Ketoconazole 110
Nefazodone 111
Nelfinavir 111
Nicardipine 111
Nifedipine 111
Posaconazole 110
Quinupristin 110
Ritonavir 111
Saquinavir 111
Telithromycin 110
Troleandomycin 110
Verapamil 111
Voriconazole 110
Vinorelbine
Amiodarone 111
Amprenavir 111
Aprepitant 111
Atazanavir 111
Clarithromycin 110
Conivaptan 111
Cyclosporine 111

<u>Underline</u> = Class 1;   *Italic* = Class 2;   Roman = Class 3

Underline = Class 1;   *Italic* = Class 2;   Roman = Class 3

Cholestyramine 27
Cimetidine 29
Colestipol 27
Co-trimoxazole 30
Danazol 31
Diclofenac 31
Dicloxacillin 27
Diflunisal 31
Disulfiram 31
Etodolac 31
Fenofibrate 31
Fenoprofen 31
Fluconazole 29
Fluorouracil 31
Fluoxetine 30
Flurbiprofen 31
Fluvastatin 28
Fluvoxamine 30
Gemfibrozil 31
Griseofulvin 27
Ibuprofen 31
Imatinib 31
Indomethacin 31
Isoniazid 31
Ketoprofen 31
Ketorolac 31
Leflunomide 31
Levothyroxine 32
Liothyronine 32
Liotrix 32
Lovastatin 28
Meclofenamate 31
Mefenamic acid 31
Mefloquine 31
Meloxicam 31
Metronidazole 30
Miconazole 29
Nabumetone 31
Nafcillin 27
Naproxen 31
Oxaprozin 31
Oxcarbazepine 27
Phenytoin 27
Piroxicam 31
Primidone 27
Propafenone 31
Rifabutin 27

Rifampin 27
Rifapentine 27
Rosuvastatin 28
St. John's Wort 27
Simvastatin 28
Sucralfate 27
Sulfamethizole 30
Sulfamethoxazole 30
Sulfaphenazole 30
<u>Sulfinpyrazone</u> 28
Sulindac 31
Tamoxifen 31
Thyroid 32
Tolmetin 31
Voriconazole 29
Zafirlukast 31
Wellbutrin. See Bupropion
Wigraine. See Ergot
Alkaloids
Xanax. See Alprazolam
Xeloda. See Capecitabine
Xenazine. See Tetrabenazine
Zafirlukast
Acenocoumarol 31
Warfarin 31
Zagam. See Sparfloxacin
Zantac. See Ranitidine
Zaroxolyn. See Metolazone
Zestril. See Lisinopril
Zidovudine
Barbiturates 112
Carbamazepine 112
Efavirenz 112
Nevirapine 112
Oxcarbazepine 112
Phenytoin 112
Primidone 112
Probenecid 112
Rifabutin 112
Rifampin 112
Rifapentine 112
St. John's Wort 112
Trimethoprim 112
Valproic acid 112
Zileuton
Clozapine 57
Olanzapine 57

Theophylline 103
Tizanidine 106
Zinc. See also Herbal
Interaction chart
Ciprofloxacin 95
Enoxacin 95
Gemifloxacin 95
Levofloxacin 95
Lomefloxacin 95
Moxifloxacin 95
Norfloxacin 95
Ofloxacin 95
Sparfloxacin 95
Tetracyclines 85
Ziprasidone. See QTc table
Zithromax. See Azithromycin
Zocor. See Simvastatin
Zolmitriptan. See also QTc
table
<u>Ergot Alkaloids</u> 70
Zoloft. See Sertraline
Zolmig. See Zolmitriptan
Zyflo. See Zileuton
Zyloprim. See Allopurinol
Zyvox. See Linezolid

<u>Underline</u> = Class 1;   *Italic* = Class 2;   Roman = Class 3

Ordering information for additional copies of
The Top 100 Drug Interactions, 2010 Edition.

Book Pricing Table:

Copies:	Price per Book
1-10	$17.95
11+	Email or call for quote

Shipping and Handling Table:

Total Order:	USA	Canada	Other Countries
<$40	$6	$8	$15
$40-75	$8	$13	$25
$76-150	$10	$17	$40
$151-300	$30	$50	$75
Over $300	Email or call	Email or call	Email or call

To mail an order, use order form on next page. For Visa MasterCard orders, go to our web site, and follow the link to "Books." Web site: *www.hanstenandhorn.com*

Phone/Fax: 360 730 1206
Email: See link at *www.hanstenandhorn.com*

H&H Publications Order Form

Hansten and Horn's
The Top 100 Drug Interactions
2010 Edition

Copies of Top 100	Price per Book	Total Book Cost
X	=	
Shipping/handling (see Table previous page)		
Sum (Total book cost plus shipping/handling)		
Washington State Tax 8.9% (Sum X 0.089)		
Total amount to send with order		

Send book to:

_____ Name

_____ Address

_____ City/State/Zip

_____ Phone / Email

Mail order with payment in US funds (check or money order) to:

H&H Publications
Box 1418
Freeland, WA 98249-1418

Looking for a more detailed reference on drug interactions to complement your copy of **The Top 100 Drug Interactions**?

Hansten and Horn's Drug Interactions Analysis and Management is a complete reference on drug-drug interactions that is updated quarterly. It contains detailed information on over 2800 interactions. Using their unique classification system, the authors have assessed each interaction for its potential risk to a patient. Factors that may alter the risk of the interaction are identified. Interaction monographs include the mechanism of the interaction and summaries of primary biomedical literature describing the interaction. Practitioners are presented with safe alternatives to consider for the avoidance of the interaction. Suggestions for patient monitoring and references are also provided.

Copies can be ordered by calling:
Facts and Comparisons, Inc at 1-800-223-0554 and asking for **Hansten and Horn's Drug Interactions Analysis and Management** or see the link at *www.hanstenandhorn.com.*

HANSTEN AND HORN'S
DRUG INTERACTION PROBABILITY SCALE

The Drug Interaction Probability Scale (DIPS) is designed to assess the probability of a causal relationship between a drug interaction and an event.

Directions: Circle the appropriate answer for each question and sum the score. Use "Unknown or NA" if a) you do not have the information, or b) the question is not applicable.

---

1. Are there credible reports of this interaction in humans?
   Yes +1, No –1, Unknown or NA 0
2. Is the observed interaction consistent with the known interactive properties of the precipitant drug?   Yes +1, No –1, Unknown or NA 0
3. Is the observed interaction consistent with the known interactive properties of the object drug?   Yes +1, No –1, Unknown or NA 0
4. Is the event consistent with the known or reasonable time course of the interaction (onset and/or offset)?   Yes +1, No –1, Unknown or NA 0
5. Did the interaction remit upon dechallenge of the precipitant drug with no change in the object drug?   Yes +1, No –2, Unknown or NA 0
6. Did the interaction reappear when the precipitant drug was readministered with continued use of the object drug?   Yes +2, No –1, Unknown or NA 0
7. Are there reasonable alternative causes for the event?[a]
   Yes –1, No +1, Unknown or NA 0
8. Was the object drug detected in the blood or other fluids in concentrations consistent with the proposed interaction?   Yes +1, No 0, Unknown or NA 0
9. Was the drug interaction confirmed by any objective evidence consistent with the effects on the object drug (other than drug concentrations)?
   Yes +1, No 0, Unknown or NA 0
10. Was the reaction greater when the precipitant drug dose was increased or less when the precipitant drug dose was decreased?
   Yes +1, No –1, Unknown or NA 0

a. Consider clinical conditions, other drugs, lack of compliance, risk factors. A "NO" answer presumes that enough information was presented so that one would expect any alternative causes to be mentioned.

Total score_____	Highly Probable	>8
	Probable	5-8
	Possible	2-4
	Doubtful	<2

The Drug Interaction Probability Scale is based on the Naranjo ADR Probability Scale adapted from Naranjo CA et al. Clin Pharmacol Ther 1981;30:239. For more details see Horn JR, Hansten PD, Chan L-N. *Proposal for a New Tool to Evaluate Drug Interaction Cases*, Ann Pharmacotherapy 2007;41:674-680.